THE 21-DAY INTERMITTENT FASTING WEIGHT LOSS PLAN

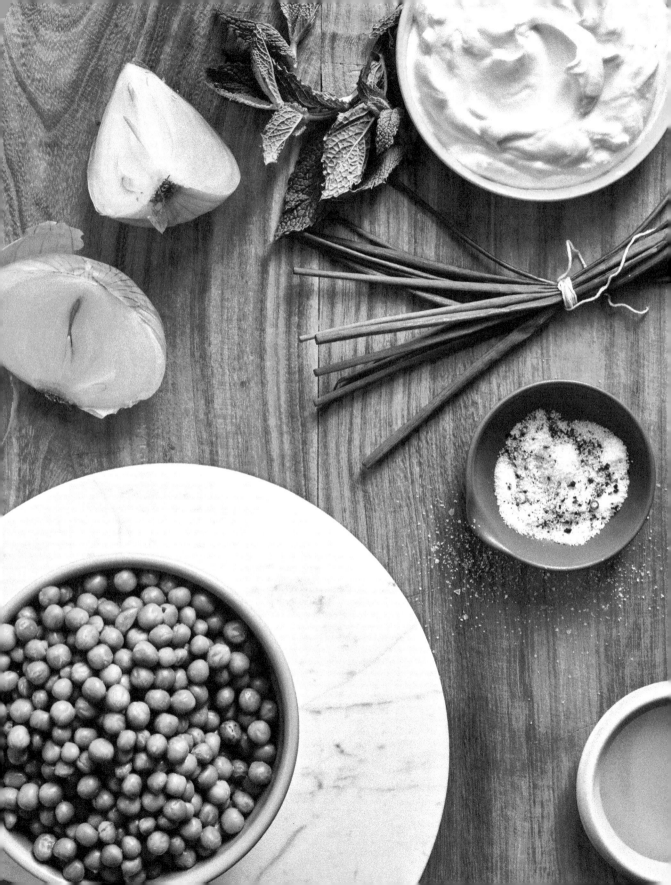

THE 21-DAY
INTERMITTENT
FASTING
WEIGHT LOSS PLAN

Recipes, Meal Plans, and Exercises for a Healthier You

ANDY DE SANTIS, RD, MPH

WITH MICHELLE ANDERSON

Photography by Biz Jones

**ROCKRIDGE
PRESS**

For general information on our other products and services or to obtain technical support, please contact our Customer Care Department within the United States at (866) 744-2665, or outside the United States at (510) 253-0500.

Rockridge Press publishes its books in a variety of electronic and print formats. Some content that appears in print may not be available in electronic books, and vice versa.

Interior and Cover Designer: Sean Doyle
Art Producer: Sara Feinstein
Editor: Laura Apperson
Photography © 2020 Biz Jones; Stocksy/Joanna Nixon, cover.
Food styling by Erika Joyce.
Illustrations 2019, 2020 © Charlie Layton
Author photo courtesy of © Natalie CD Photography.

ISBN: Print 978-1-64611-570-9 | eBook 978-1-64611-571-6
R0

This book required a great deal of research and scientific referencing to write, and my lovely lady, Rebecca, made the formatting of those references easy for me with her help and expertise.
Thanks, Bec!

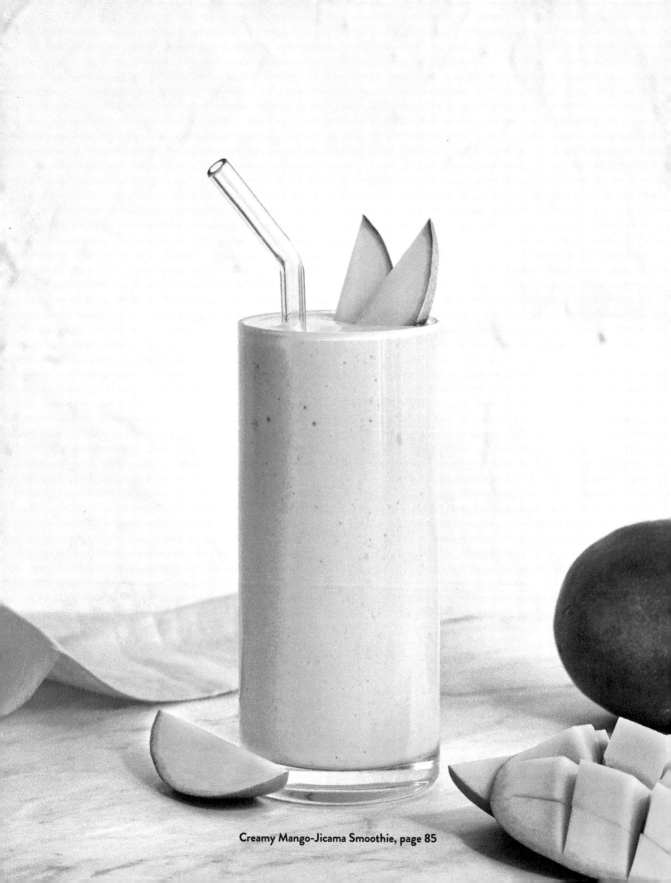

Creamy Mango-Jicama Smoothie, page 85

Contents

Welcome to the 21-Day Plan

"The best of all medicines are rest and fasting."
–Benjamin Franklin

WELCOME TO YOUR THRILLING JOURNEY into the world of intermittent fasting!

As a registered dietitian and a general food nut, intermittent fasting has become an integral part of both my personal and professional lives.

I've greatly enjoyed experimenting and implementing various types of fasts into my own routine, studying all the available evidence behind fasting, and bringing all that knowledge to my clients.

Today, I am fortunate enough to be writing my fourth book, one I hope will help people understand the health benefits of intermittent fasting. This book is arguably the one that I was most excited to write given my absolute passion for intermittent fasting. So, when I say that I can't wait to embark on this journey with you, I mean that genuinely.

What I love about intermittent fasting more than anything else is that it has helped me enjoy my meals. I was very active in my twenties, and I ate whatever I wanted, as much as I wanted, whenever I wanted. Once my work-life balance shifted after age 30, my metabolism inevitably did as well, and I found myself wholly unable to keep eating the same way I did when I was younger. I'm sure this story sounds familiar to you so far.

I enjoyed eating larger meals, so this new reality really bothered me. I found myself lacking the hunger I used to have and simply could not enjoy meals like I used to. That's what drew me to intermittent fasting. I did things in a flexible manner and on my terms, which is the style of fasting I offer you in the pages to come. The guidance in this book is not gimmicky or dogmatic; rather, it is a pragmatic, real-life approach to fasting that is aimed at optimizing both enjoyment and weight-loss results.

As much as I am guilty of jumping on the proverbial bandwagon, it's hard not to chuckle at the recent surge in popularity of fasting when you consider the fact that it has existed in historical and religious contexts for ages. Famous Greek philosophers such as Hippocrates and Plato were noted to have been interested in fasting, while the famous Swiss physician Paracelsus was quoted in the 1500s as saying, "Fasting is the greatest remedy—the physician within."

So, on that note, let's embark on the path to releasing your "physician within." This book introduces everything you need to know and more about the art and science of intermittent fasting. It presents an expertly crafted 21-day plan to put you on the path toward your weight-loss goals and help you seamlessly embrace fasting.

Let's get started.

PART I

THE INTERMITTENT FASTING PLAN

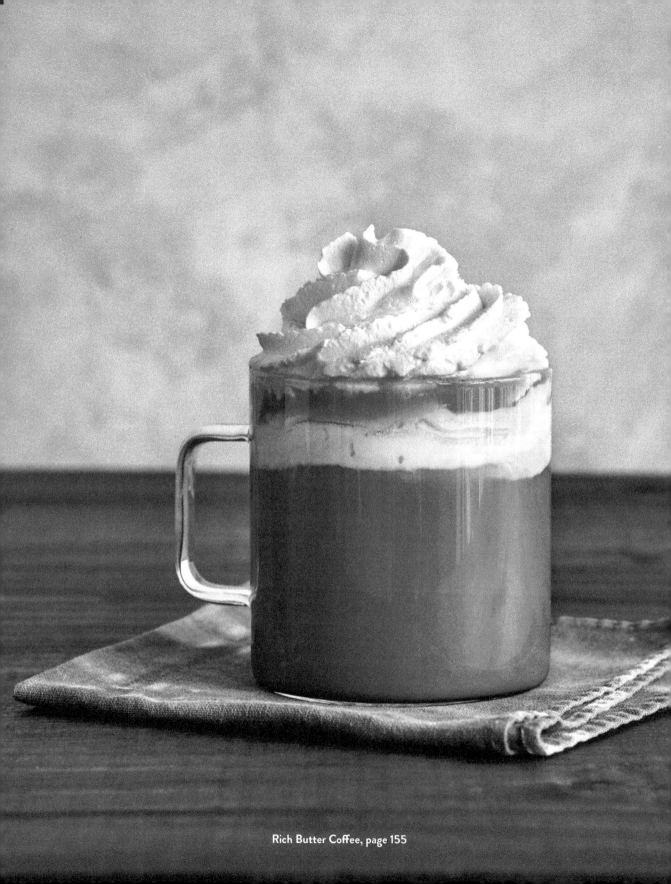

Rich Butter Coffee, page 155

CHAPTER 1

LOSING WEIGHT WITH INTERMITTENT FASTING

INTERMITTENT FASTING is one of the most popular and effective tools I've used in my practice to support my clients' weight-loss goals.

In this chapter, we cover what intermittent fasting is, why it works, and why I'm so confident that once you start, you will wonder what took you so long to give it a try.

What Is Intermittent Fasting?

Intermittent fasting is a broadly encompassing term that involves an intentional manipulation of the length of time one goes without eating. You might pursue intermittent fasting for a variety of reasons, ranging from convenience, to lifestyle preferences, to health, to weight loss. Intermittent fasting asks these two very basic questions:

1. What is the length of time from your last bite of food one day to your first bite the next?

2. Are you willing to extend that window? How often and by how much?

Your answers will shape what intermittent fasting means to you, which will likely evolve with time, self-awareness, and experience. Most types of intermittent fasting do not explicitly tell you what you can or cannot eat; rather, you're required to think more about timing when you structure your meals on any given day. While the recipes provided in part 2 have been expertly crafted to guide you toward healthier eating, they will not artificially restrict you from any given food group.

So, can just modifying the timing of your meals really have that great of an effect on your health? Both history and modern science think so. Various forms of intermittent fasting have been practiced throughout human history across a broad range of civilizations for both medical and religious reasons.

Some daring folks even engage in extended fasts, which involve abstaining from food for multiple days at a time. These types of fasts are extreme in nature, and although they may be enjoyed by a very limited number of people, they are not particularly appealing to most, nor are they necessary to achieve the benefits associated with fasting. With that in mind, prolonged multiday fasts are not discussed in this book.

Instead, we will concentrate on six daily and weekly intermittent fasting styles, which include fasts ranging from 12 to 24 hours in duration. Let's take a closer look at our options.

TYPES OF INTERMITTENT FASTING

In this section, you will gain a better understanding of the different types of intermittent fasting options at your disposal, including an explanation of the differences between daily and weekly fasts, and all the subtypes within these two groups.

When helping clients who are interested in fasting determine the type of intermittent fast that's best for them, my philosophy is simple: We change fasting to fit your life; we don't change your life to fit fasting. In other words, you do not need to turn your social and professional life upside down to fit an arbitrary fasting regimen. Fasting is supposed to make your life easier and more enjoyable.

DAILY FASTS

Daily fasts are, obviously, carried out on a daily or near-daily basis. The number designations relate to the window of time to be spent either eating or fasting. Those who are new to fasting or are wanting to ease into it are free to conduct any of the following daily fasts on alternate days, rather than every day, as they see fit.

12:12

A 12:12 fast is the lightest possible version of intermittent fasting. On this fast, leave a 12-hour window from your last bite one day until your first bite the next day. For example, if you finish eating at 7 p.m., you can eat your next meal at 7 a.m. the next day.

This fast serves as a great initial entry point for individuals who are concerned about how they might respond to intermittent fasting or for those who simply are not yet interested in going without food longer than 12 hours.

16:8

The 16:8 style of fasting is the most commonly implemented fast. This fast allows a 16-hour period from the last bite one day to the first bite the next, designating an 8-hour "eating window." For example, if you finish eating at 7 p.m., you can eat your next meal at 11 a.m. the next day. It's a simple and logical progression from the 12:12 fast that can be eased into using a 14:10 style of fasting as an intermediary step if preferred.

ONE MEAL A DAY (OMAD)

One meal a day (OMAD) is a simple way to describe what would ultimately be close to a 22:2, 23:1, or even 24:0 fast, where you would eat a single large meal after having gone at least 22 hours without eating. If you finished eating at 7 p.m. one night, you'd likely wait a full day and eat your next meal between 5 p.m. and 7 p.m. The OMAD-style of fasting is more likely to be used in a more dynamic fashion—once in a while—and not as a hard-and-fast daily rule. This is considered an advanced daily fast.

WEEKLY FASTS

Weekly fasts differ from daily fasts in that you may be engaging in fasting only a few days a week, but on those days, you may be required to pay a little more attention to how many calories you eat. That really depends on how you choose to carry it out, so let's take a closer look at the options, which progress in difficulty.

5:2

In the 5:2 fast, you eat normally five days of the week but fast with a lowered calorie intake—between 500 and 800 calories—the other two days. These calories can be consumed in a single, large meal or two smaller meals or snacks.

Alternatively, a gentler version of a 5:2 fast would require a normal diet five days per week followed by a 16-hour fast two days a week without the explicit calorie restriction.

ALTERNATE-DAY MODIFIED FASTING (ADMF)

Alternate-day modified fasting, or ADMF, alternates between days of eating freely and days of calorie-controlled fasting. On calorie-controlled fasting days, you'd eat between 500 and 800 calories over one to two meals or snacks, which may end up looking like a calorie-controlled version of 16:8. It is a more involved version of the 5:2 fast because you end up calorie-controlled fasting three to four days per week rather than just two.

ALTERNATE-DAY FASTING (ADF)

Alternate-day fasting, or ADF, could also be thought of as 1:1 fasting, because it involves a repeated cycle of eating freely one day and fasting completely the next. This is probably the most advanced and challenging style of fasting that will be discussed in the book. A milder version of alternate-day fasting could involve implementing a daily fast, such as 16:8, every other day.

BUSTING FASTING MYTHS

The recent increase in fasting's notoriety brings with it some detractors. However, in 2017, the journal *Annual Review of Nutrition* noted that "evidence suggests that intermittent fasting regimens are not harmful physically or mentally (i.e., in terms of mood) in healthy adults."

This section will separate fact from fiction when it comes to some of the myths around intermittent fasting.

Myth #1: Fasting is starving. Going a bit longer between meals does not equate to starvation. Starvation is a scientifically defined state where your body has burned much of its fat and glycogen reserves and resorts to protein (in other words, muscle) to use for fuel. No types of fasting described in this book are intended to fling your body into the depths of "starvation" mode.

Myth #2: Fasting deprives you of nutrients. If someone just decided to start fasting on a whim without a deeper consideration of their overall dietary pattern, it is possible they could fall short on certain nutrients. That won't happen to anyone reading this book; as long as you understand the meals you are most likely to miss and account for foods that comprise those meals elsewhere in your day, your risk of nutrient inadequacy is incredibly low.

Myth #3: Fasting leads to overeating. It's very likely that, when fasting, you could end up eating larger and less frequent meals. But if you define overeating from a caloric perspective, it's not likely to occur with a well-planned fasting program. In fact, a 2017 article from *Annual Review of Nutrition* claims that weight loss can occur through almost any intermittent fasting regimen.

How Men and Women Fast Differently

One of the underpinnings of scientific thought around intermittent fasting is that it puts the human body under low levels of stress but ultimately makes it more resilient. You could almost think of it as a workout regimen for your metabolism.

While this continues to be of great interest to researchers, we are left to grapple with how to approach fasting as a potential stressor, especially considering how men and women react differently to stress both psychologically and biologically, as examined by a 2009 study reported in the journal *Endocrine Disorders*, which found that women tend to have higher circulating levels of the stress hormone cortisol.

Cortisol is not the only hormonal difference between men and women, though. The interaction between intermittent fasting and menstruation is another relevant consideration for women.

To address this question, we can look to data from the fasting month of Ramadan. Ramadan replicates a daily intermittent fast of between 12 and 16 hours and offers relevant insights applicable to other types of fasting. In a 2013 Ramadan-based study, the *Iranian Journal of Reproductive Medicine* reported that menstrual abnormalities increased, especially in women fasting for 15 or more days straight. One in 10 participants had menstrual abnormalities before Ramadan, but that number rose to 3 in 10 during Ramadan.

Looking at these numbers, it is certainly a relevant consideration, particularly for those with a history of menstrual abnormalities.

From the hormonal perspective, another Ramadan-based study published in 2014 in the *Clinical and Experimental Obstetrics and Gynecology* journal found important female hormones, including luteinizing hormone, follicle-stimulating hormone, and estradiol, all remained within normal ranges throughout the month-long fast.

Taking all the data into consideration, there is no reason for women to be fearful of intermittent fasting, even if it is advisable that they pay an extra bit of attention to how their bodies respond to it.

WHO CAN AND CANNOT FAST?

The vast majority of available evidence suggests that, for otherwise healthy adults, fasting is safe both mentally and physically.

Although I've incorporated different levels of intermittent fasting successfully with people from all walks of life and nutritional backgrounds, I'm under no impression that fasting is a one-size-fits-all solution. Some people are comfortable only with shorter fasts, while others don't mind the lengthier ones. Others should not be fasting at all. My number one rule for fasting is that if it is not improving your quality of life, you probably should not be doing it.

Those with medical conditions, either acute or chronic, should consult a doctor before fasting. Although intermittent fasting is almost always carried out with the goal of improving one's health, there are instances when it could be dangerous, or at the very least unadvisable.

These cases include:

History of eating disorders. Some styles of intermittent fasting may partially mimic or resemble restrictive styles of eating, which could trigger those with a history of disordered eating or food restriction.

Pregnant/breastfeeding. Women who are pregnant or breastfeeding have higher caloric needs than others, and adequate nutrient intake for the health of themselves and their child takes priority.

Underweight/undernourished. Although intermittent fasting is not solely a weight-loss tool, certain styles lend themselves to eating fewer calories. Fasting is not recommended for anyone underweight or with nutrient inadequacies.

Specific medications. Certain medications are contingent on the consumption of varying amounts of foods, and fasting should not take precedence over the scheduled intake of these medications without consulting a health-care professional.

Children and teenagers. Young people are at a stage of rapid growth and development and have extremely high-calorie and nutrient needs. The regular inclusion of fasting regimens could interfere with those needs.

How Intermittent Fasting Aids in Weight Loss

For those who are healthy, willing, and able, intermittent fasting offers a unique approach to weight loss that provides benefits through two specific paths, practical and metabolic.

THE PRACTICAL PATH

The practical path to weight loss through intermittent fasting relies on the notion that intermittent fasting is a strategic and comfortable way to consume fewer calories. Anyone who is engaging in a prolonged and regular intermittent fasting regimen will consume fewer calories than they used to, simply because there is less time in the day allotted for eating. When combining a shorter eating window with more filling and satisfying choices, like the ones found in this book, the potential for losing weight is certainly there. This assertion is supported by the findings of a 2018 study in the journal *Nutrition and Healthy Aging*, which found that fasting led to mild calorie reduction without the need to count or monitor caloric intake.

THE METABOLIC PATH

The metabolic path suggests that through fasting you gain unique metabolic advantages that support weight loss. Consistently going for extended periods of time without food has a beneficial effect on human metabolism, which a growing body of scientific evidence seems to support.

According to a 2015 study from the *Rejuvenation Research* journal, intermittent fasting alters the expression of genes related to human metabolism and longevity. The long-term effects of such alterations require further research to confirm, but they are certainly of great interest.

Multiple studies, including the one previously cited, a 2017 review paper from the *Behavioural Sciences* journal, and a 2018 paper in *Cell Metabolism*, have demonstrated intermittent fasting to have either a superior effect on circulating insulin levels or insulin resistance, as compared to "normal dieting." Bodily insulin resistance can develop with age and poor dietary habits, leading to higher blood sugar levels because your liver and muscle cells become less inclined to take up and process circulating sugars. According to a 2005 paper from one of the American Heart Association journals, insulin is a major driver of fat cell storage, which means that higher levels of circulating insulin may stimulate an increase in fatty tissue and contribute to weight gain.

Some scientists also believe that fasting offers additional weight-loss benefits because it improves the efficiency of the energy-processing mechanisms in your body, forcing them to be more flexible in the face of prolonged periods without food. This phenomenon, known as metabolic flexibility, may have some role to play in the benefits associated with intermittent fasting, although more research is needed in this area to draw firm conclusions.

WHAT HAPPENS WHEN YOU FAST?

Have you ever wondered what metabolic changes take place when you fast? This section will explain this by breaking fasting down into three stages.

Nowhere does this book prescribe a style of fasting that requires going any longer than 24 to 36 hours without food, so we keep the descriptions within those parameters.

Stage 1: The Fed State (First 3 hours after last meal)

An increase in blood glucose from your last meal leads to insulin secretion. The use of fat as fuel is inhibited, and your body uses available carbohydrates for energy, storage, or both. Excess energy intake may be stored as fat.

Stage 2: The Early Fasting State (3 to 18 hours after last meal)

Your insulin and blood sugar levels normalize, and your body now relies on glycogen stores in the liver for energy. As more time passes, your body will switch to breaking down fat for energy.

Stage 3: The Fasting State (18 to 36 hours after last meal)

Building from stage 2, your metabolism begins to shift into primarily using fat as a fuel source with the risk of muscle breakdown increasing, especially beyond the 36-hour period.

Fasting and the Hunger Hormone

Hormones are signaling molecules that effect different types of change throughout the body.

The beneficial effects of fasting on hormone levels represent a sort of extension of the metabolic path, but the link between intermittent fasting and hormones goes beyond just insulin—the hormone that moves glucose into your cells to be used as energy.

Let's consider ghrelin, which is aptly named the "hunger hormone" because it is strongly associated with appetite and tends to be at its highest levels right before a meal. A 2019 study in the journal *Obesity* looked at women engaged in an 18:6 fasting regimen, a slightly more advanced version of the 16:8 described in this book. The researchers found that despite being engaged in a lengthy daily fast, the women's appetite levels decreased and their hunger was more even-keeled throughout the day. The kicker? Their hunger hormone levels decreased, too.

Although fasting theoretically increases your hunger in the short term, in the intermediate term, it may help you be more in touch with whether or not you are actually hungry.

Achieving Your Weight Loss Goals with the 21-Day Plan

Intermittent fasting is an incredibly valuable tool to power you on the path toward your goals, but it must be applied strategically in conjunction with a healthy diet to ensure success.

HEALTHIER EATING WHILE FASTING

The 21-day plan and the nutritious recipes in part 2 will be your guide to healthy eating while fasting. The recipes take a clean-eating approach, focusing on dietary pillars such as fruits, vegetables, nuts, seeds, legumes, whole grains, fish, and lean meats. A diet emphasizing these foods is nourishing, filling, and metabolically stimulating, which is why the recipes have been created with these pillars in mind.

One of the things I love about intermittent fasting for weight management is that it does not artificially restrict any large groups of foods, which is a breath of fresh air! Such is the power of manipulating the timing and scheduling of when you eat; you are actually granted quite a bit more freedom than when dieting. Many diets tell you what you can't eat, rather than focusing on the wonderful things you can.

In the next section, I will more fully explain why the foods you eat—not the foods you avoid—determine your success both over the next 21 days, and what I hope will be a lifelong journey using both healthy eating and intermittent fasting.

CALORIES, FULLNESS, AND FASTING

Success with intermittent fasting is contingent upon eating meals that are equal parts delicious and satiating. Most beginner-friendly styles of intermittent fasting rely on the metabolic benefits of fasting, the reduction in overall food consumption and calories that come with a shorter eating window, and the effects of higher protein intake.

One of the real perks of intermittent fasting is that, for the most part, you don't need to be hyper-focused on your caloric intake. Rather than calorie tracking, fasting relies on a shortened eating window, sufficient protein intake, and a modest boost to your metabolism to support weight loss.

There are certainly some exceptions, like during weekly fasts when you are asked to keep your intake within a specific range. I also appreciate that you might need some guidance on calorie recommendations to support your weight-loss goals. Although exact calorie requirements to support weight loss vary widely from person to person depending on factors such as age, gender, and activity level, I will simplify things for you as much as possible.

The average calorie range to support weight loss in most men is between 1,750 to 2,250 calories per day. Men who are under 50 and more active will be on the higher end of that range, whereas men who are over 50 and less active will be on the lower end.

The average calorie range to support weight loss in most women is between 1,250 and 1,750 calories per day. Women who are under 50 and more active will be on the higher end of that range, whereas women who are over 50 and less active will be on the lower end.

For reference, if you are fasting purely for lifestyle and general health benefits and not weight loss, your recommended calorie levels will be closer to 2,250 to 2,750 calories per day for men and 1,750 to 2,250 calories per day for women. Those who are so inclined can use these values to guide their overall consumption patterns in conjunction with the meal plans provided. It's important to keep in mind that the meal plans offer you a guide, but that the total number of calories will vary slightly depending on the day, the style of fast you choose, and the amount of each recipe you choose to consume.

In most cases, having only a single serving of each of the recipes offered will not provide enough calories for the day. This will allow you to incorporate snacks or increase the suggested serving size of your meal as you see fit. Feel free to double—or maybe halve—serving sizes, depending on your calorie needs and whether you are planning on replacing a lunch recommendation with leftovers from dinner.

Let's take a minute to talk more about the importance of protein. The recommended daily allowance for protein intake is set at 0.8 g/kg (grams per kilogram), but multiple studies have shown there are additional metabolic benefits when protein intake is increased by a minimum of 50 percent, closer to 1.2 g/kg per day, and even up to 1.6 g/kg and beyond. This is especially true for those engaged in regular resistance training.

At this level of protein intake, satiety tends to be greater and the potential for weight loss is higher, at least partially due to what is known as the thermic effect of food, meaning it takes more energy for your body to break down protein than either carbohydrates or fat. A 2017 study in the *Obesity Facts* journal found that individuals who consumed the same number of calories but more protein (1.34 g/kg per day versus 0.8 g/kg per day) experienced greater weight loss. There is also a better chance for muscle mass retention during weight loss when protein intake is higher, which is a very important consideration for athletes and active people.

With these facts in mind, the emphasis for those engaging in the 12:12, 16:8, or even OMAD fasts will just be good old-fashioned healthy eating with plenty of protein and fiber. For the 5:2 and ADMF, your intake is limited to 500 to 800 calories. On these more challenging fasting days, an emphasis on high protein and fiber intake will be all the more important.

Conventionally, we think of high-protein foods as chicken, eggs, beef, and dairy, whereas high-fiber foods are usually thought of as fruits and veggies. It's very rare that a whole food be high in both protein and fiber, yet these particular foods are gems when it comes to both fasting and healthy eating in general.

The most prominent and underrated foods in this category, which also happen to be extremely affordable, are legumes: black beans, lentils, chickpeas, kidney beans, and so on. One cup of legumes, on average, has a whopping 17.5 grams of both fiber *and* protein. No other food boasts such high amounts of both, in addition to a plethora of vitamins, minerals, and antioxidants, all in one place.

POSITIVE THINKING AND REACHING YOUR GOALS

As with all things related to health and nutrition, the manner in which you frame things can play a very large role in determining your success. This is especially true when fasting, especially for those who are new to it. Remember, you have opted to give fasting a shot because you want to, not because you have to.

With that in mind, how will you choose to look at the last few hours of a daily fast? Will you frame it positively by looking forward to how much you will enjoy your first meal of the day? This type of thinking is conducive to intermittent fasting success, especially the more challenging styles.

Intermittent fasting is intrinsically reward-driven because we all love to eat, but the biggest mistake I see clients make is getting too caught up in the structure and not listening to their body's cues.

For example, let's say someone is doing an alternate-day 16:8 fast and they wake up ravenous on a fasting day. Should they still fast? I say absolutely not.

The same could be said about waking up quite full to the point of discomfort on a nonfasting day. Why wouldn't you consider fasting?

Because so many of us eat in a ceremonial fashion at specific times each day, we sometimes lose touch with whether or not we are actually hungry. Remember that intermittent fasting is an intuitive and dynamic tool that takes time to master, just as any other skill would. Ultimately, placing your emphasis on enjoying the process, rather than focusing only on the outcome, is going to put you in a much better position to succeed.

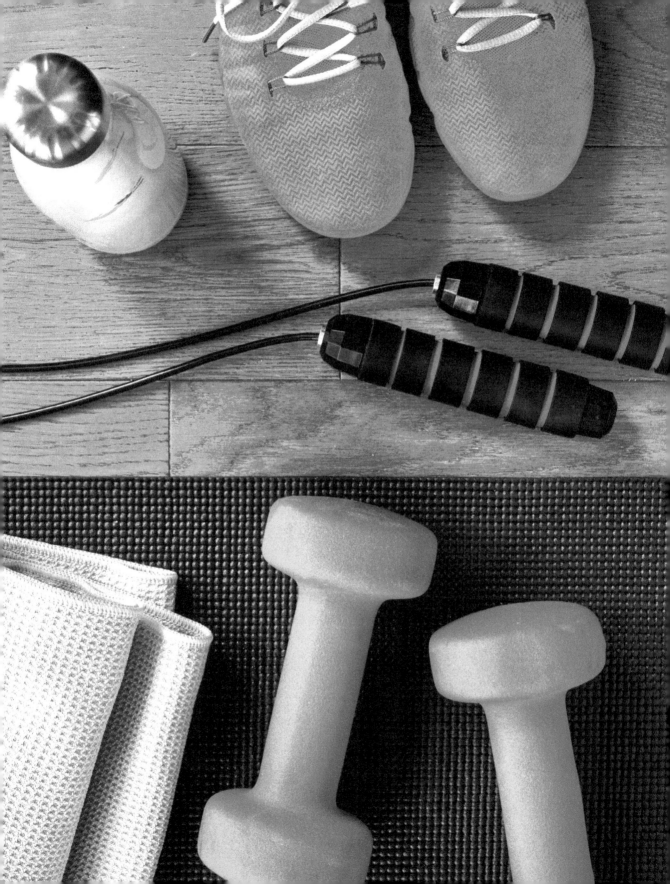

CHAPTER 2

PLANNING YOUR EXERCISE

THIS CHAPTER INTRODUCES the exercises that will make up the workout portion of your 21-day plan and shows you how to combine intermittent fasting and physical activity in a way that works for you.

Exercise During Your Fast

Let's start by differentiating working out while fasting versus working out while fasted.

Working out while fasting simply means incorporating regular physical activity into your routine while also engaging in some sort of fasting regimen. For example, you could be practicing 16:8 and choose to always work out after you break your fast.

Working out while fasted refers specifically to engaging in physical activity while in the fasted state, having not eaten for an extended period of time. Working out while fasted is not for everyone. Some of my clients do it without thinking twice, while others can't stand the thought. That's totally fine—your comfort comes first.

It's very important to choose a fasting and exercise routine that works for you, which might take a bit of experimentation. The next few sections will point you in the right direction.

ADJUSTING TO YOUR FASTING BODY

How you adjust to regular intermittent fasting depends on a number of factors, including your previous experience with fasting, the regimen you're following, and the full picture of your current diet and exercise routine. Individual preferences and comfort levels also come into play. If you are new to fasting, it might take your body time to adapt.

Longer fasts or prolonged fasting days may, for some people, be less conducive to good workouts while fasted—but that doesn't necessarily have to be the case. Don't be too concerned if, at the end of a long fast, you don't feel up for an intense workout; that's quite normal. No matter which angle you're coming at this from, keep the following tips in mind.

STAY HYDRATED

Adequate hydration is critical for you to thrive and perform whether you are fasting or not. As you adapt to fasting, however, it's that much more important to confidently check the hydration box. The recommended water intake, as set by the Institute of Medicine in 2005, is about 2.7 L (91 oz.) a day for women and 3.7 L (125 oz.) per day for men. One cup of water is 250 mL, or 8.5 oz. Technically, this recommendation also includes water provided from all foods and beverages.

Drinking enough water and other fluids may play a small role in keeping you satiated during your fast, but I do not recommend consuming excessive amounts of water in an attempt to combat hunger. If you are that hungry, it's time to break the fast.

Fasting is not supposed to be torturous, and it's perfectly acceptable to break a fast early or not fast at all on a day your body just does not agree with it.

CAFFEINE HELPS

Caffeine happens to be one of the most studied naturally occurring performance boosters. It enhances alertness, reduces perceptions of fatigue, and may give you that preworkout boost you need in the early stages of fasting adaptation. Although caffeinated beverages like coffee and tea can encourage you to consume more total daily fluids, it won't make or break your intermittent fasting success. So, don't sweat it if you aren't a regular caffeine consumer.

TAKE YOUR FOOD SERIOUSLY

It probably won't surprise you to hear this coming from a dietitian, but it's very important not to underestimate the value of healthy, balanced eating while engaging in any sort of intermittent fasting routine. Optimal fiber, protein, and overall nutrient intake is fundamental for not only satiation but also for physical and exercise performance.

EXPERIMENT WITH YOUR APPROACH

I'm a firm believer that intermittent fasting is a skill, and skills take time to master. You may not arrive on the right type of fasting or the optimal exercise routine on your first attempt, but don't let that stop you. Some people may notice a big difference in how they feel working out on a fasting day as opposed to working out at the end of that same day. You don't know until you try, so let's take a closer look at how you can ease toward establishing a routine that works for you.

ESTABLISHING A ROUTINE

In the next chapter, you will choose the fasting plan that works for you; in this section, you will be encouraged to think about how exercise might fit into that plan. Physical activity usually spans three broad categories: strength, endurance, and mobility. Strength is gained through resistance training, endurance through cardiovascular activity, and mobility through activities like yoga and stretching. A balanced exercise routine makes considerations for all of the preceding; how they fit into your routine is ultimately up to you, and the movements provided in this chapter will certainly help. If you intended to work out seven days per week, for example, you might devote three to strength, three to endurance, and at least one to mobility, stretching, and recovery, which could also be implemented on the other days.

Ask yourself, *Am I open to working out on a fasted day?* Many of my clients, as a matter of personal preference and comfort, choose to fast on days they don't plan to exert themselves too much physically. This is especially true of morning exercisers.

That leads to the next question, *Do I intend to exercise in the morning or evening?* Usually, people have a hard-and-fast preference and comfort level with the time of day they work out, and I don't expect or want you to change that. You should adjust fasting to fit your life, not your life to fit fasting.

Let's use the very common 16:8 style of fasting to exemplify this point. In my experience, most people opt to fast from the evening to morning. In that case, a 16:8 fast would involve not eating between the hours of 8 p.m. and noon. That gives the average person working a 9-to-5 job three distinct options, each with limitations:

1. **Morning workout.** This approach could increase your appetite and make it harder to fast, although this is less of an issue for daily fasts of moderate length.

2. **Late-afternoon workout.** This is potentially the most physically challenging because you are at the peak of fast duration, though you will certainly enjoy breaking your fast more than usual.

3. **Late-evening workout.** This allows for working out in a well-fed state but is not always practical due to timing constraints and may involve exercise with more food in your stomach than you'd prefer. It could also interfere with sleep patterns.

There are pros and cons to each approach. It really comes down to comfort, safety, and personal preference.

Workouts That Don't Feel Like Workouts

If the usual multimove routine or 30-minute run just isn't speaking to you one day, try something else. Activities like soccer, basketball, tennis, rock climbing, swimming, jumping rope, and biking all burn some serious calories. Also, don't be too quick to underestimate how much energy your body expends doing more strenuous household activities like mowing the lawn, chopping wood, or shoveling the snow. Beyond the workout routines offered in this book, there are endless at-home routines, from yoga to martial arts, that will really spice up the way you think about fitness.

Intermittent Fasting for Athletes

Athletes may train while fasted for metabolic benefits or perhaps even for the challenge of it. However, athletes have above-average energy needs, and their performance depends on optimal fueling before, during, and after training and competition.

A 2012 paper from the *Journal of Sports Sciences* that looked at athletes who fasted during Ramadan, which is very similar to a 16:8 daily fast, helps makes sense of this apparent disparity, and suggests that as long as diet quality and quantity remain sufficient, there is little risk to performance in fasting athletes.

Looking more specifically at performance in a fed versus fasted state, a 2018 study in the *Scandinavian Journal of Medicine & Science in Sports* found that eating before exercise makes for better performance in aerobic exercise lasting 60 minutes or longer but has no significant effect on shorter durations of activity. The study also found potential metabolic benefits of training while fasted, including the enhanced use of fat for fuel in the post-exercise period.

Based on my review of the preceding evidence, strategic intermittent fasting could fit into the training regimens of most athletes as long as there was a desire to do so and proper attention is paid to the overall quantity and quality of food intake.

Cardio and Bodyweight Exercises

A diverse workout program emphasizing both cardiovascular and strength training exercises will represent an integral component of your 21-day plan. Allotting a minimum period of about 30 minutes most days to engage in some form of physical activity is a reasonable way to approach this plan.

Your strength training routine will be comprehensive, including movements focusing on the core, lower body, and upper body, as well as some full-body exercises. We've selected moves that will challenge you but can be done at home without requiring much equipment beyond some dumbbells, a mat, and a bench.

CARDIO

BRISK WALKING. Walk at a rate faster than your normal walking pace for getting from point A to point B.

RUNNING. Working toward longer and more intense runs is a great way to build cardiovascular fitness.

JOGGING. Jogging is the intermediary stage between brisk walking and running and can be used as an accompaniment to either exercise, depending on your fitness level.

JUMPING JACKS. Jumping jacks are best practiced as a complement to other cardio exercises on this list.

DANCING. Anyone can put on their favorite music and dance like there's nobody watching. There are also a number of online dance workouts and programs at your disposal if you are so inclined.

JUMP ROPE. Jumping rope is a fun way to get your heart rate up and is much harder than it looks.

OTHER OPTIONS (EQUIPMENT PERMITTING). Consider other activities such as rowing, swimming and water aerobics, biking, yoga, and using elliptical and stair climbing machines for a great workout.

CORE

PLANK. The plank is the quintessential core exercise that focuses on stability and strength of the muscles in the abdominal and surrounding areas. While facedown, engage your buttocks and press your forearms into the ground, holding for 60 seconds. If you are a beginner to this pose, consider starting with a 15- to 30-second hold and work your way up.

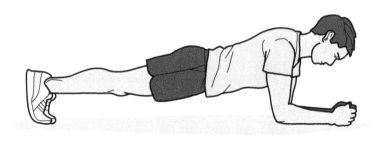

SIDE PLANK. Another fundamental movement, this plank variation focuses on the oblique muscles on either side of your central abdominals. Make sure your torso does not sag toward the ground and keep the buttocks tight.

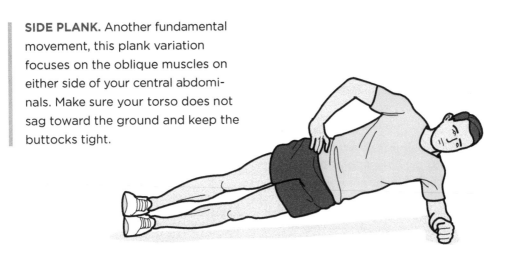

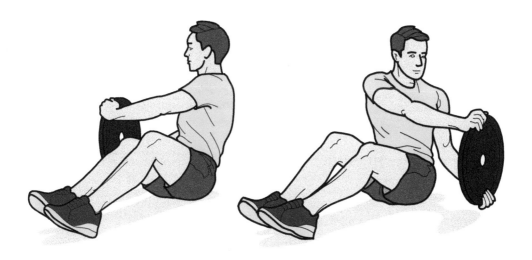

RUSSIAN TWIST. Sitting on your bottom, keep your chest up, shoulders back, back flat with your feet a few inches off the floor, and lean back slightly. Hold a weight plate or dumbbell at waist height, and twist your torso right to left, pausing a few seconds at each end point.

LOWER BODY

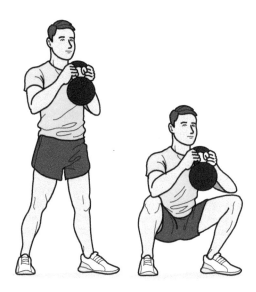

GOBLET SQUAT. Place your feet a little wider than shoulder-width apart and hold a dumbbell tightly with both hands in front of your chest. Gently move down into a squat, taking care to hinge at both the knee and the hip joints, and lower your legs until they are parallel to the ground. Using your heels, move back up to the starting position and repeat. Use a chair to squat onto if necessary for balance.

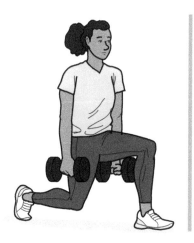

DUMBBELL WALKING LUNGE. Start in the same position as the goblet squat—feet a little wider than shoulder-width apart—but without weights. With one leg, step forward and sink down until your back knee is just above the ground. Check to be sure the front knee is not bending over your toes and keep your torso tall and upright. Push through the heel of the front foot and step forward and through with your rear foot. Add one or two dumbbells as you feel comfortable. Looking for more of a challenge? Switch your walking lunge to a jump lunge without the weights.

ROMANIAN DEAD LIFT. Different from the squat and lunge, this exercise focuses on the hamstrings, which are your leg's rear muscles. Start in a walking lunge position, except be sure to hinge at the hips and push your buttocks and hips backward while naturally lowering the dumbbells in front of you. As you ascend back to the starting position, squeeze your buttocks. You can also do this exercise on one leg, which improves your balance and activates your core, but use lighter weights.

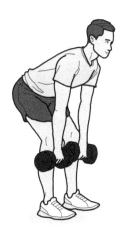

UPPER BODY

PUSH-UPS. Push-ups are a fantastic exercise that require no equipment. Lie facedown with your hands just beyond shoulder-width apart, keeping your body in a straight line and engaging your core as you ascend and descend. Don't let your elbows flare out. Beginners can start by performing them on their knees or even against a wall.

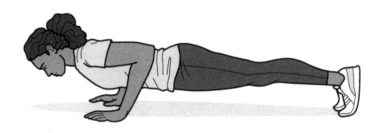

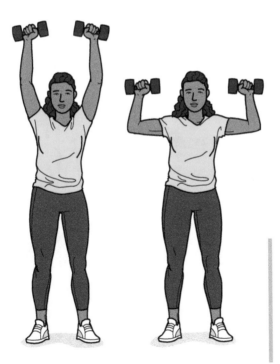

DUMBBELL SHOULDER PRESS. A great exercise for upper body and shoulder strength that is more challenging than it looks. Hold one dumbbell in each hand and bring them to ear level with palms forward and then straighten arms overhead.

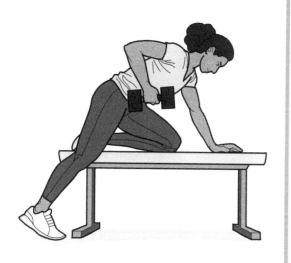

SINGLE-ARM DUMBBELL ROWS.
This popular exercise improves the strength of your back muscles. Place your left knee and hand on an exercise bench or other flat, firm surface. With a flat back, eyes forward, and palms facing in, hold the dumbbell with your right hand and raise it up, taking care to keep your elbow tucked into your side. Hold and contract for up to two seconds, then release back to where you started. Reverse sides. Want to spice up the routine? A more challenging alternative that works some of the same muscle groups is pull-ups.

FULL BODY

MOUNTAIN CLIMBER. Position your body in a plank, with your abdominal and buttocks muscles engaged. In quick succession, alternate pulling your knees into your chest while keeping your core engaged. Continue in this left, right, left, right knee rhythm as if you are replicating a running motion. Keep your spine in a straight line.

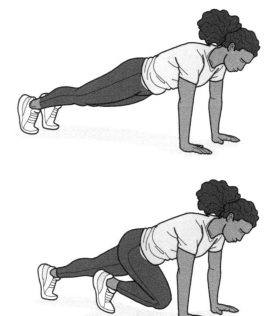

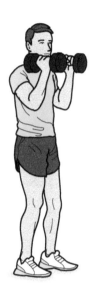
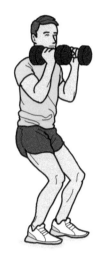
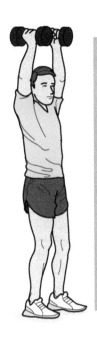

PUSH PRESS. This move incorporates both a partial squat and a dumbbell shoulder press. Using a comfortable weight, place your feet slightly wider than shoulder-width apart, with dumbbells held a little lower than your ears. Move down into a comfortable squat, and as you come back up, push the dumbbells overhead.

BURPEE (OPTIONAL). This is an advanced, dynamic exercise that combines a push-up, a squat, and a jump. It is very effective but challenging and should be used only by those who feel able. Start from a standing position, with feet slightly wider than shoulder-width apart, before lowering into a squat, placing your hands on the floor. Jump backward to land on the balls of your feet into a plank position while keeping your core strong. Jump back to your hands and jump again into the air, reaching your hands upward. Want more of a challenge? Jump higher and tuck your knees if you can.

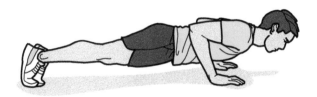

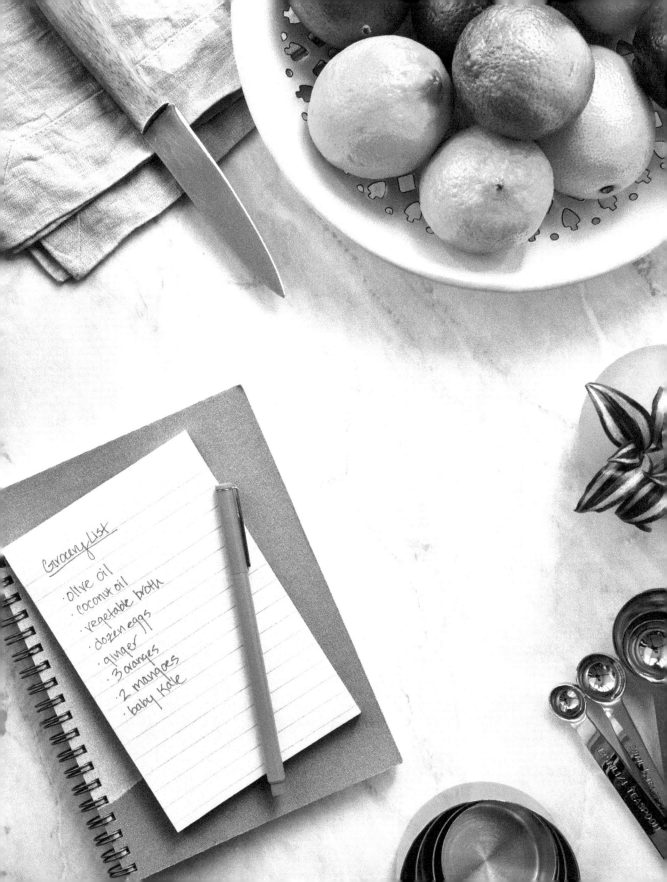

Grocery List

- olive oil
- coconut oil
- vegetable broth
- dozen eggs
- ginger
- 3 oranges
- 2 mangoes
- baby kale

CHAPTER 3

YOUR 21-DAY PLAN

GET READY to bring your 21-day plan to life; it will play an important role in setting you on your path to success with intermittent fasting. It's not all or nothing though. Each week is unique and specifically customized to the six styles of fasting discussed in the book. If you start with a type of fast that does not work for you in week 1, you have the freedom to shift your plan to a different fast in weeks 2 and 3.

Pantry, Refrigerator, and Freezer Staples

Before we dive into week 1 and all the good stuff that comes with it, I'll outline some dietary essentials that have a big role in the 21 days ahead of you. These staples are required to make every meal in the book, but you won't necessarily need to buy everything at once. Before you make your shopping list for each week, consider how many people you are cooking for besides yourself, how many leftovers you might have (if any), and how many calories you need to consume for your selected fast. Keep in mind that if you have leftovers from one meal, you can refrigerate or freeze them and replace another meal in the plan with those leftovers.

PANTRY ESSENTIALS

Healthy Fats

- Avocado
- Butter
- Coconut
- Coconut oil
- Nuts and nut butters: almonds, cashews, peanuts, pecans, pistachios, walnuts, and so on
- Olive oil
- Olives
- Seeds: chia, flax, hemp, pepita, pumpkin, sesame, sunflower, and so on
- Sesame oil
- Tahini

Beans and Legumes

- Black beans
- Chickpeas
- Kidney beans
- Lentils
- Navy beans

Whole Grains

- Barley
- Buckwheat
- Bulgur
- Farro
- Noodles: chow mein, soba
- Oats
- Quinoa
- Rice: brown, wild, and so on

Herbs and Spices

- Basil
- Bay leaves
- Chili powder
- Chives
- Cilantro
- Cinnamon
- Coriander
- Cumin
- Curry powder
- Dill
- Fennel
- Garlic/garlic powder
- Ginger
- Mint
- Nutmeg
- Oregano
- Paprika
- Parsley
- Pepper
- Red pepper flakes
- Sea salt
- Thyme

Sweeteners

- Honey
- Maple syrup
- Molasses
- Pure vanilla extract

Other

- Baking powder
- Baking soda
- Cajun seasoning
- Cayenne pepper
- Cloves
- Cocoa powder
- Coffee
- Cooking spray
- Corn taco shells
- Dijon mustard
- Flours/alternative flours: almond flour, cornstarch, and so on
- Hoisin sauce
- Hot chili oil
- Miso
- Oyster sauce
- Protein powder
- Soy sauce alternatives: tamari sauce or coconut aminos
- Tea: green
- Unsweetened nut/ seed butters: almond butter, peanut butter, sunflower seed butter, and so on
- Vinegars: apple cider, balsamic, rice, white wine
- Whole-grain or multigrain bread
- Whole-wheat pitas
- Whole-wheat tortillas
- Worcestershire sauce

REFRIGERATOR AND FREEZER ESSENTIALS

Fruit

- Apple
- Apple juice
- Applesauce
- Banana
- Berries: blackberries, blueberries, raspberries, strawberries, and so on
- Cherries
- Dates
- Lemon
- Lime
- Mango
- Nectarine
- Oranges
- Peach
- Pear

Vegetables

- Artichoke hearts
- Asparagus
- Bean sprouts
- Bok choy
- Broccoli
- Cabbage: red, green, Napa
- Cauliflower
- Celeriac
- Celery
- Corn
- Cucumber
- Edamame
- Eggplant
- Fennel
- Green beans
- Green peas
- Greens: chard, collard greens, kale, mustard greens, spinach, and so on
- Jalapeño
- Jicama
- Leeks
- Lettuce
- Mushrooms: portobello
- Onions: yellow, sweet, and red
- Peppers: green, yellow, orange, and red
- Pumpkin
- Radishes
- Root vegetables: beets, carrots, parsnips, potatoes, sweet potatoes, and so on
- Scallions
- Snow peas
- Squash: acorn squash, butternut squash, and so on
- Tomatoes: cherry, diced, crushed, paste, stewed
- Zucchini

Meats and Proteins

- Beef: ground beef
- Canadian bacon
- Eggs
- Pork
- Poultry: chicken, turkey, and so on
- Shellfish and freshwater fish: shrimp, haddock, trout, salmon, and so on
- Tofu

Dairy and Dairy Alternative Products

- Buttermilk
- Cheese: blue cheese, feta, Parmesan, ricotta
- Cottage cheese
- Kefir
- Milk
- Milk alternatives: almond, cashew, coconut, oat, rice, soy, and so on
- Sour cream
- Yogurt/Greek yogurt

Fast-Friendly Items

Technically speaking, your caloric intake should be as close to zero as possible during a fast. This means you will rely primarily on water, carbonated water, tea, and black coffee for hydration during the fasting period. Plain beef, chicken, and other types of broths are also acceptable, very low-calorie options during a fast. Ideally, you will keep caloric intake from beverages as low as possible during a fast, so look for choices in the 25- to 50-calorie range.

Chapter 10 will provide more elaborate broth and beverage recipes that are slightly higher in calories than what one might include during a strict fast, but they will play an important role for beginners and those testing out longer fasts. Feel free to rely on these items at your discretion with the knowledge that they technically break your fast but could be useful, especially during the first of the three weeks.

How to Choose and Meal-Plan Your Fasting Method

The most important thing to take away from this section is that fasting is meant to be modified to fit your life. In other words, you should not have to turn your personal and social life upside down to fit a specific style of intermittent fasting. I never expect this of my clients, and I certainly do not expect it of you. Although short-term progress is relevant, true success always comes in the medium to long term, and I can't stress enough how important it is for you to keep that in mind as you venture forward on this fasting journey.

As we head into the next section where we will cover meals plans for the different types of fasts, start asking yourself these important questions:

- What time of day do I prefer to do most of my eating?

- Do I prefer frequent, more modest fasts or infrequent, longer ones?

- Is there a time of the week more conducive to fasting?

I will also offer as many alternative strategies as possible to ensure that you arrive at a style of fasting, or perhaps a combination of styles, that works best for you.

DAILY FASTS

Daily fasts can be carried out in one of two ways: every day, as the name suggests, or on alternate days—especially for those who find it practically challenging to commit to daily fasting. For example, if fasting 12 hours a day seems like too much to start, you can always ease into it by doing it every other day.

An alternate daily fast is not to be confused with ADF (alternate-day fasting), which is actually considered a weekly fast.

12:12

The 12:12 daily fast is a gentle introduction to intermittent fasting. Most people will be able to pull off this style of fasting by eating as they usually would throughout the day and cutting out evening snacking. This fast requires a 12-hour period from your last bite at night to your first bite the next day. For example, if you finish around 7:30 p.m. and have breakfast the next day at around 7:30 a.m., you've successfully completed a 12-hour fast. If you are a person who does not reach for the healthiest stuff late in the evening, this style of fasting will be beneficial.

While it may be the shortest type of fasting recommended in this book, it still counts and makes for a great entry point and stepping-stone to longer fasts.

16:8

The 16:8 fast is for those who have either outgrown a 12:12 fast or feel that 12:12 fasting is too similar to what they already do. Keep in mind that if the jump from 12:12 to 16:8 feels daunting, you can always use a 14:10 fasting period as an intermediary step, in which you fast for 14 hours from your last bite one day to your first bite the next.

There are a number of ways to carry out a 16:8 fast, but most people do so by eating only between the hours of noon and 8 p.m. This means that in addition to omitting evening snacking, you are omitting your first meals and snacks of the day and carrying on your day from there once your fasting period is over.

Some people erroneously describe 16:8 fasting as nothing more than just "skipping breakfast." That's a bit of an oversimplification because you could technically eat traditional breakfast food, such as a yogurt parfait, for lunch.

Some people will also opt to carry out what is known as the "early time-restricted feeding" (ETRF) version of this fast, meaning they will eat for an 8-hour period starting early in the morning (6 a.m. to 9 a.m.) and finish in the late afternoon (2 p.m. to 5 p.m.). In this case, you'd be omitting your final meal of the day. If you want to try a 16:8 fast and prefer to eat more at the beginning of the day than the end, or you just absolutely love a big breakfast at home, it may be ideal for you.

ONE MEAL A DAY (OMAD)

The OMAD-style of fasting appeals to those who really enjoy eating large meals and can't be bothered to think about food all day. The biggest advantage is that you have complete freedom from worrying about if/what/when you will eat. However, some people may find the hunger associated with this type of fasting hard to bear.

Certain types of healthy foods such as nuts and seeds usually aren't regularly consumed as part of meals, but more so as snacks. Therefore, if you eat only one meal per day, you may find yourself omitting these types of foods. Beware of this and be sure your meals day-to-day and week-to-week include a wide variety of foods, including healthy snacks and breakfast items, to ensure variety and nutritional adequacy in your diet.

WEEKLY FASTS

During a weekly fast, you won't fast on a daily basis. When it is time to fast, the duration tends to be longer.

5:2

Traditionally, 5:2 weekly fasting refers to eating on a normal schedule for five days of the week, then consuming only about 500 to 800 calories the other two days. This generally amounts to either a single meal or two snacks, as per your preference.

It may be helpful to think of those two fasting days as somewhere between 16:8 and OMAD with extra attention paid to your overall caloric intake. This is different from daily fasts, where you do not have to actively monitor your caloric intake. The two fasting days do not need to be carried out back-to-back and can be spread out to make them more manageable.

Beginners to fasting who are not ready for daily or alternating daily fasts could also technically use those two "fasting days" to incorporate a 16:8 fast without the caloric restriction. This is a very reasonable entry point for those who may feel overwhelmed by the idea of regular or intense fasts.

This style of fasting may appeal to people who are naturally less hungry on certain days of the week, perhaps because they are more likely to eat out, or eat more the day prior.

ALTERNATE-DAY MODIFIED FASTING (ADMF)

If you are a more proficient faster who has mastered a 5:2 style of fasting and want to expand your repertoire, you might consider trying alternate-day modified fasting (ADMF). ADMF is a slightly less extreme version of alternate-day fasting because you consume 500 to 800 calories on fasting days. The ADMF fast is actually the midpoint between 5:2 and alternate-day fasting since you fast with a calorie restriction between three and four days a week as part of your routine. This is considered an advanced fast.

ALTERNATE-DAY FASTING (ADF)

Alternate-day fasting (ADF) is the most challenging of all fasting regimens. You really have to enjoy fasting to even consider it. ADF is not to be confused with alternating daily fasts, which are simply engaging in a certain style of fasting (such as 16:8) every other day. Alternate-day fasting is quite different and entails eating freely one day but abstaining from food fully the next.

Presumably, most people attempting this type of fasting will consume additional or larger meals or snacks on nonfasting days and are drawn to the idea of fasting fully the next day. In terms of meal planning, an individual attempting ADF has a number of options at their disposal, such as including an extra daily snack or doubling up on the size of their dinner on eating days.

Week 1

I tell my clients you have to take one step before you can take two, so I congratulate you as you prepare to embark on your first step: week 1. Week 1 is all about adaptation, new beginnings, and the element of the unknown. You want to try fasting in a structured way for the first time, or you may be dabbling in a new type of fasting.

For all types of fasting meal plans and further specific instructions are provided. I encourage you to listen to your body and be honest about how you're feeling. Don't be afraid to miss a day or switch to a lighter style of fasting if you feel you need to.

DAILY FASTS

This section provides a customized meal plan and instructions for each of the three types of daily fasts. In addition to recipe recommendations, each plan considers the unique nature of each fasting style to make the process that much easier for you.

12:12

FASTING TIME	12 hours
EATING TIME	12 hours
CALORIES ALLOWED DURING FAST	None
MEALS PER DAY	3 meals per day, snacks optional

The meal plan provided for 12:12 fasters will be very much business as usual, incorporating healthy recipes for breakfast, lunch, and dinner. Feel free to replace any lunch recommendation with leftovers from dinner.

The flexibility of 12:12 allows for a very routine day of eating with the goal of a 12-hour fasting period from your last bite one day to your first bite the next.

	BREAKFAST	LUNCH	DINNER
SUNDAY	Baked Cinnamon-Orange French Toast	Broccoli-Beef Stir-Fry with Black Bean Sauce	Classic Roasted Vegetables with Nutmeg
MONDAY	Mixed Grain Porridge with Pear & Maple	Skillet Asian Chicken Breasts	Hearty Turkey-Vegetable Stew
TUESDAY	Ricotta-Oatmeal Pancakes	Wild Rice–Spinach Stew	Kale-Beef Rolls
WEDNESDAY	Spicy Panzanella Breakfast Casserole	Beef-&-Farro-Stuffed Peppers	Pecan-Tofu Noodle Salad
THURSDAY	Blueberry–Green Tea Smoothie	Chicken & Sweet Potato with Peaches	Market Bulgur-Chicken Skillet
FRIDAY	Avocado, Roasted Red Pepper & Tofu Scramble	Parsnip–Sweet Potato Frittata	Black Bean & Sun-Dried Tomato Quesadillas
SATURDAY	Shrimp-Kale Omelet	Rustic Beef & Cabbage Stew	Mediterranean Fish Tacos

FASTING TIME	16 hours
EATING TIME	8 hours
CALORIES ALLOWED DURING FAST	None
MEALS PER DAY	2 meals per day, snacks optional *Note:* Beginners may choose to fast only on alternating days.

The meal plans provided for 16:8 fasters will only include lunch and dinner to facilitate the 16-hour fasting period.

Depending on your usual routine, you may also choose to incorporate a snack either in between or after these meals or increase the serving size of the meal, especially during the first week or two. Feel free to replace any lunch recommendation with leftovers from dinner.

If you are planning on doing early time-restricted feeding (ETRF), you will want to consume breakfast and lunch but omit dinner, in which case you can follow the breakfast recipes allotted for the 12:12 plan.

Remember, the key component here is the 16-hour period from your last bite one day to your first bite the next.

	BREAKFAST	LUNCH	DINNER
SUNDAY	FAST	Broccoli-Beef Stir-Fry with Black Bean Sauce	Classic Roasted Vegetables with Nutmeg
MONDAY	FAST	Skillet Asian Chicken Breasts	Hearty Turkey-Vegetable Stew
TUESDAY	FAST	Wild Rice–Spinach Stew	Kale-Beef Rolls
WEDNESDAY	FAST	Beef-&-Farro-Stuffed Peppers	Pecan-Tofu Noodle Salad
THURSDAY	FAST	Chicken & Sweet Potato with Peaches	Market Bulgur-Chicken Skillet
FRIDAY	FAST	Parsnip–Sweet Potato Frittata	Black Bean & Sun-Dried Tomato Quesadillas
SATURDAY	FAST	Rustic Beef & Cabbage Stew	Mediterranean Fish Tacos

FASTING TIME	22 to 23 hours
EATING TIME	1 to 2 hours
CALORIES ALLOWED DURING FAST	None
MEALS PER DAY	1 large meal per day *Note:* Remember to adjust the serving size for your one meal to eat all your normal daily calories and add any supplemental snacks to ensure you are getting all your nutrients.

Guess what you're getting for OMAD? One meal. Most people engaging in OMAD will opt just to eat dinner, so that is the recipe that is provided. Because you are relying on a single meal a day to meet your calorie and nutrient needs, you will likely need to consume multiple servings of any recipe provided and potentially combine it with other foods, or even additional recipes, as you see fit. If you regularly engage in OMAD-style fasting, it's imperative to ensure sufficient variety in your meals from day-to-day so that you don't miss out on important nutrients in the long term. If you find yourself unbearably hungry during the day or struggling for variety in your diet with an OMAD routine, you may consider extending your eating window so that you can incorporate a second meal or snack to address either or both of those concerns.

This is also a great opportunity to head to chapter 10 and explore some of the fast-friendly broths and beverages at your disposal.

	BREAKFAST	LUNCH	DINNER
SUNDAY	FAST	FAST	Classic Roasted Vegetables with Nutmeg
MONDAY	FAST	FAST	Hearty Turkey-Vegetable Stew
TUESDAY	FAST	FAST	Kale-Beef Rolls
WEDNESDAY	FAST	FAST	Pecan-Tofu Noodle Salad
THURSDAY	FAST	FAST	Market Bulgur-Chicken Skillet
FRIDAY	FAST	FAST	Black Bean & Sun-Dried Tomato Quesadillas
SATURDAY	FAST	FAST	Mediterranean Fish Tacos

WEEKLY FASTS

This section provides a customized meal plan and special instructions for each of the three types of daily fasts discussed in this book. In addition to recipe recommendations of what to cook and eat on a given day, each plan comes with insights that consider the unique nature of each fasting style with the goal of making the process that much easier for you.

5:2

FASTING DAYS PER WEEK	2
NORMAL EATING DAYS PER WEEK	5
CALORIES ALLOWED DURING FASTING DAYS	<800
MEALS PER DAY	All calories are eaten within 1 to 8 hours on fasting days, either in one sitting on fasting days *or* in two smaller meals.

On normal days, 5:2 fasters will follow the standard plans of three meals per day for a given week.

On fasted days, you will consume between 500 and 800 calories in a 16:8 or OMAD fasting regimen.

If you intend to follow the meal plan provided, note the calories per serving so that you can have a better understanding of your daily total.

You may also choose to eat differently and focus on snacks or smaller meals on fasting days, in which case some additional effort is required to ensure you stay within the 500- to 800-calorie range. You might, for example, choose to eat one large meal in the 500- to 800-calorie range, or if you prefer to spread it out, you might have one moderately sized meal and one snack of about 300 calories to land you in that range.

For days you are not fasting, feel free to replace any lunch recommendation with leftovers from dinner.

	BREAKFAST	LUNCH	DINNER
SUNDAY	Baked Cinnamon-Orange French Toast	Broccoli-Beef Stir-Fry with Black Bean Sauce	Classic Roasted Vegetables with Nutmeg
MONDAY	FAST	Skillet Asian Chicken Breasts	Hearty Turkey-Vegetable Stew
TUESDAY	Ricotta-Oatmeal Pancakes	Wild Rice–Spinach Stew	Kale-Beef Rolls
WEDNESDAY	Spicy Panzanella Breakfast Casserole	Beef-&-Farro-Stuffed Peppers	Pecan-Tofu Noodle Salad
THURSDAY	FAST	Chicken & Sweet Potato with Peaches	Market Bulgur-Chicken Skillet
FRIDAY	Avocado, Roasted Red Pepper & Tofu Scramble	Parsnip–Sweet Potato Frittata	Black Bean & Sun-Dried Tomato Quesadillas
SATURDAY	Shrimp-Kale Omelet	Rustic Beef & Cabbage Stew	Mediterranean Fish Tacos

ALTERNATE-DAY MODIFIED

FASTING DAYS PER WEEK	3 to 4
NORMAL EATING DAYS PER WEEK	3 to 4
CALORIES ALLOWED DURING FAST	<800
MEALS PER DAY	All calories are eaten in within 1 to 8 hours on fasting days, either in one sitting on fasting days *or* two smaller meals. *Note:* Because alternating days can mean you fast either 3 or 4 days in a week, you can alter the difficulty of the fast by choosing whether the first day of the week is a fasting or eating day.

Alternate-day modified fasters will follow the standard weekly plan every other day and consume 500 to 800 calories on either a 16:8 or OMAD regimen the other days of the week. If you intend to follow the meal plan provided, note the calories per serving so that you can have a better understanding of your daily total. You may also choose to eat differently and focus on snacks or smaller meals on fasting days, in which case some additional effort is required to ensure you stay within the 500- to 800-calorie range. You might choose to eat one large meal in the 500- to 800-calorie range, or if you prefer to spread it out, you might have one moderately sized meal and one snack of about 300 calories to land you in that range.

For days you are not fasting, feel free to replace any lunch recommendation with leftovers from dinner.

	BREAKFAST	LUNCH	DINNER
SUNDAY	Baked Cinnamon-Orange French Toast	Broccoli-Beef Stir-Fry with Black Bean Sauce	Classic Roasted Vegetables with Nutmeg
MONDAY	FAST	Skillet Asian Chicken Breasts	Hearty Turkey-Vegetable Stew
TUESDAY	Ricotta-Oatmeal Pancakes	Wild Rice–Spinach Stew	Kale-Beef Rolls
WEDNESDAY	FAST	Beef-&-Farro-Stuffed Peppers	Pecan-Tofu Noodle Salad
THURSDAY	Blueberry–Green Tea Smoothie	Chicken & Sweet Potato with Peaches	Market Bulgur-Chicken Skillet
FRIDAY	FAST	Parsnip–Sweet Potato Frittata	Black Bean & Sun-Dried Tomato Quesadillas
SATURDAY	Shrimp-Kale Omelet	Rustic Beef & Cabbage Stew	Mediterranean Fish Tacos

FASTING DAYS PER WEEK	3 to 4 *Note:* Full day of fasting on alternating days
NORMAL EATING DAYS PER WEEK	3 to 4 *Note:* Full day of eating on alternating days
CALORIES ALLOWED DURING FAST	None
MEALS PER DAY	3 meals per day on eating days, snacks optional, none on fasting days *Note:* Because alternating days can mean you fast either 3 or 4 days in a week, you can alter the difficulty of the fast by choosing whether the first day of the week is a fasting or eating day.

Alternate-day fasters will eat freely one day and fast the next. On free-eating days you can use the following meal plan provided. You may choose to incorporate additional snacks or double the serving size of certain recipes as your hunger dictates.

For days you are not fasting, feel free to replace any lunch recommendation with leftovers from dinner.

	BREAKFAST	LUNCH	DINNER
SUNDAY	Baked Cinnamon-Orange French Toast	Broccoli-Beef Stir-Fry with Black Bean Sauce	Classic Roasted Vegetables with Nutmeg
MONDAY	FAST	FAST	FAST
TUESDAY	Ricotta-Oatmeal Pancakes	Wild Rice–Spinach Stew	Kale-Beef Rolls
WEDNESDAY	FAST	FAST	FAST
THURSDAY	Blueberry–Green Tea Smoothie	Chicken & Sweet Potato with Peaches	Market Bulgur-Chicken Skillet
FRIDAY	FAST	FAST	FAST
SATURDAY	Shrimp-Kale Omelet	Rustic Beef & Cabbage Stew	Mediterranean Fish Tacos

YOUR EXERCISE ROUTINE

Cardio workouts should be 30 minutes in duration, but you can work up to that if you are a beginner. Strength workouts should generally include three to four sets of 8 to 10 repetitions of each exercise where applicable. In the case of static core exercises, such as the plank, work toward holding the move longer each week.

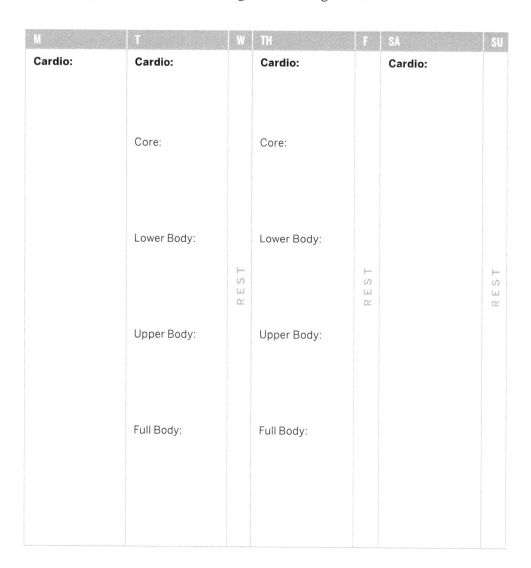

M	T	W	TH	F	SA	SU
Cardio:	**Cardio:**	REST	**Cardio:**	REST	**Cardio:**	REST
	Core:		Core:			
	Lower Body:		Lower Body:			
	Upper Body:		Upper Body:			
	Full Body:		Full Body:			

WELLNESS TRACKER

The wellness tracker is an optional but very useful tool to keep tabs on some of the important health behaviors that are encouraged in this book.

Your overall fasting duration, drinking enough water, sleeping eight hours a night, and eating multiple servings of fruits and vegetables are all very important habits you could choose to track using this helpful tool.

HABIT	M	T	W	TH	F	SA	SU
DRINK 8 GLASSES OF WATER	X		X			X	X

Week 2

Welcome to week 2! A delicious new combination of recipes awaits!

Week 2 is all about learning, reflecting, and modifying based on your experience in week 1.

Did you enjoy the style of fasting you chose? If not, I hope you gained valuable insight into which style of fasting may be a better fit. Don't be afraid to modify your fasting style or try a different one altogether. In the big picture, one week will not dictate much. The same goes for your workouts.

In week 2 you are treated to a brand-new meal plan with all-new recipes from top to bottom. My bet is that you are starting to enjoy your post-fast meals more than your usual meals, and I expect that to continue for the next seven days.

DAILY FASTS

This section provides a customized meal plan and special instructions for each of the three types of daily fasts discussed in the book.

12:12

FASTING TIME	12 hours
EATING TIME	12 hours
CALORIES ALLOWED DURING FAST	None
MEALS PER DAY	3 meals per day, snacks optional

If you are starting your second week of 12:12, that means the first went well and you want to keep at it. For those who feel comfortable, I'd encourage slightly extending your fast on a few days of the week to maybe 13 or 14 hours, just to test it out. If you are new to 12:12 because a different style of fasting was perhaps too much for you, I recommend referring to the 12:12 section from week 1 for further guidance.

Remember, you can feel free to replace any lunch recommendation with leftovers from dinner.

	BREAKFAST	LUNCH	DINNER
SUNDAY	Classic Eggs & Canadian Bacon	Traditional Falafel Pockets	Chopped Chicken– Brown Rice Salad
MONDAY	Date-Fennel Smoothie	Baked Chicken Breasts with Butternut Squash–Pear Salsa	Roasted Pork Chops with Chickpea– Cherry Tomato Salsa
TUESDAY	Mixed Grain Porridge with Pear & Maple	Market Bulgur- Chicken Skillet	Pearl Barley– Turkey Soup
WEDNESDAY	Fruit & Nut Yogurt Parfait	Rich Pork Stroganoff	Broiled Beef Tenderloin with Maple Barbecue Sauce
THURSDAY	Creamy Mango– Jicama Smoothie	Pumpkin-Kale Tortilla Wraps	Salmon–Navy Bean Salad
FRIDAY	Almond Butter– Quinoa Smoothie	Honey Sesame Salmon with Bok Choy	Rich Pork Stroganoff
SATURDAY	Baked Egg & Herb Portobello Mushrooms	Pork Tenderloin Medallions with Herb Sauce	Cajun-Style Fish Tomato Stew

16:8

FASTING TIME	16 hours
EATING TIME	8 hours
CALORIES ALLOWED DURING FAST	None
MEALS PER DAY	2 meals per day, snacks optional *Note:* Beginners may choose to fast only on alternating days.

If this is your second week of 16:8, congratulations! If you are here graduating from 12:12 or perhaps taking a step back from a more robust fast, welcome! Don't forget you have the option of slightly shortening the fast to 14:10 or extending to 18:6 in this second week.

For those of you who were more conservative with your physical activity in week 1 as you adjusted to your fast, considering ramping it up in week 2 if you're comfortable doing so.

Feel free to replace any lunch recommendation with leftovers from dinner.

	BREAKFAST	LUNCH	DINNER
SUNDAY	FAST	Traditional Falafel Pockets	Chopped Chicken–Brown Rice Salad
MONDAY	FAST	Baked Chicken Breasts with Butternut Squash–Pear Salsa	Roasted Pork Chops with Chickpea–Cherry Tomato Salsa
TUESDAY	FAST	Market Bulgur-Chicken Skillet	Pearl Barley–Turkey Soup
WEDNESDAY	FAST	Rich Pork Stroganoff	Broiled Beef Tenderloin with Maple Barbecue Sauce
THURSDAY	FAST	Pumpkin-Kale Tortilla Wraps	Salmon–Navy Bean Salad
FRIDAY	FAST	Honey Sesame Salmon with Bok Choy	Rich Pork Stroganoff
SATURDAY	FAST	Pork Tenderloin Medallions with Herb Sauce	Cajun-Style Fish Tomato Stew

OMAD

FASTING TIME	22 to 23 hours
EATING TIME	1 to 2 hours
CALORIES ALLOWED DURING FAST	None
MEALS PER DAY	1 large meal per day *Note:* Remember to adjust the serving size for your one meal to reach all your normal daily calories and add any supplemental snacks to ensure you are getting all your nutrients.

If you tried OMAD during week 1, you probably have some idea of whether it's a good fit for you. Remember, you always have the option of shortening your fasting period, switching to a different style of fasting, or simply doing OMAD a few days rather than every day of the week. Refer to week 1 for further guidance if you are aiming to try OMAD for the first time in week 2.

	BREAKFAST	LUNCH	DINNER
SUNDAY	FAST	FAST	Chopped Chicken–Brown Rice Salad
MONDAY	FAST	FAST	Roasted Pork Chops with Chickpea–Cherry Tomato Salsa
TUESDAY	FAST	FAST	Pearl Barley–Turkey Soup
WEDNESDAY	FAST	FAST	Broiled Beef Tenderloin with Maple Barbecue Sauce
THURSDAY	FAST	FAST	Salmon–Navy Bean Salad
FRIDAY	FAST	FAST	Rich Pork Stroganoff
SATURDAY	FAST	FAST	Cajun-Style Fish Tomato Stew

WEEKLY FASTS

This section provides a customized meal plan and special instructions for each of the three types of weekly fasts discussed in the book.

5:2

FASTING DAYS PER WEEK	2
NORMAL EATING DAYS PER WEEK	5
CALORIES ALLOWED DURING FASTING DAYS	<800
MEALS PER DAY	All calories are eaten in within 1 to 8 hours on fasting days, either in one sitting on fasting days *or* two smaller meals.

If you are coming back to 5:2 fasting after a successful first week, welcome back! Remember, it's very important to make your meals count on your fasting days; consume plenty of protein and fiber within your calorie limit to keep you full and satisfied. For days that you are not fasting, feel free to replace any lunch recommendation with leftovers from dinner.

If you found 5:2 a bit too much, I'd recommend switching over to a 16:8 daily fast. If you found it too easy and want to take things to the next level, ADMF is your best bet.

If you're trying 5:2 for the first time this week, refer to the guidance provided in week 1 for more details.

	BREAKFAST	LUNCH	DINNER
SUNDAY	Classic Eggs & Canadian Bacon	Traditional Falafel Pockets	Chopped Chicken–Brown Rice Salad
MONDAY	FAST	Baked Chicken Breasts with Butternut Squash–Pear Salsa	Roasted Pork Chops with Chickpea–Cherry Tomato Salsa
TUESDAY	Mixed Grain Porridge with Pear & Maple	Market Bulgur-Chicken Skillet	Pearl Barley–Turkey Soup
WEDNESDAY	Fruit & Nut Yogurt Parfait	Rich Pork Stroganoff	Broiled Beef Tenderloin with Maple Barbecue Sauce
THURSDAY	FAST	Pumpkin-Kale Tortilla Wraps	Salmon–Navy Bean Salad
FRIDAY	Almond Butter–Quinoa Smoothie	Honey Sesame Salmon with Bok Choy	Rich Pork Stroganoff
SATURDAY	Baked Egg & Herb Portobello Mushrooms	Pork Tenderloin Medallions with Herb Sauce	Cajun-Style Fish Tomato Stew

ALTERNATE-DAY MODIFIED

FASTING DAYS PER WEEK	3 to 4
NORMAL EATING DAYS PER WEEK	3 to 4
CALORIES ALLOWED DURING FAST	<800
MEALS PER DAY	All calories are eaten in within 1 to 8 hours on fasting days, either in one sitting on fasting days *or* two smaller meals. *Note:* Because alternating days can mean you fast either 3 or 4 days in a week, you can alter the difficulty of the fast by choosing whether the first day of the week is a fasting or eating day.

Welcome to week 2 of ADMF! I appreciate that going three days a week with a calorie limit can be challenging, so if you found it a bit too much, don't hesitate to consider trying 5:2 or allowing yourself 250 more calories on fasting days to make things more enjoyable. Don't forget to emphasize protein and fiber-rich meals, especially on fasting days. For days you are not fasting, feel free to replace any lunch recommendation with leftovers from dinner.

If you are an experienced faster looking for a challenge beyond ADMF, alternate day fasting is your best choice.

If you are new to ADMF this week, please refer to the detailed instructions in week 1.

	BREAKFAST	LUNCH	DINNER
SUNDAY	Classic Eggs & Canadian Bacon	Traditional Falafel Pockets	Chopped Chicken–Brown Rice Salad
MONDAY	FAST	Baked Chicken Breast with Butternut Squash–Pear Salsa	Roasted Pork Chops with Chickpea–Cherry Tomato Salsa
TUESDAY	Mixed Grain Porridge with Pear & Maple	Market Bulgur-Chicken Skillet	Pearl Barley–Turkey Soup
WEDNESDAY	FAST	Rich Pork Stroganoff	Broiled Beef Tenderloin with Maple Barbecue Sauce
THURSDAY	Creamy Mango–Jicama Smoothie	Pumpkin-Kale Tortilla Wraps	Salmon–Navy Bean Salad
FRIDAY	FAST	Honey Sesame Salmon with Bok Choy	Rich Pork Stroganoff
SATURDAY	Baked Egg & Herb Portobello Mushroom	Pork Tenderloin Medallions with Herb Sauce	Cajun-Style Fish Tomato Stew

FASTING DAYS PER WEEK	3 to 4 *Note:* Full day fasted on alternating days
NORMAL EATING DAYS PER WEEK	3 to 4 *Note:* Full day of eating on alternating days
CALORIES ALLOWED DURING FAST	None
MEALS PER DAY	3 meals per day on eating days, snacks optional, none on fasting days *Note:* Because alternating days can mean you fast either 3 or 4 days in a week, you can alter the difficulty of the fast by choosing whether the first day of the week is a fasting or eating day.

Welcome to week 2 of what is arguably the most challenging fasting style discussed in this book. If going without food on alternating days proved too daunting, consider trying ADMF or 5:2, both of which allow you to consume calories on fasting days.

If you are new to alternate-day fasting, be sure to review the guidance offered in week 1, and do not hesitate to break a fast if you need to.

Remember that for days you are not fasting, you can replace any lunch recommendation with leftovers from dinner.

	BREAKFAST	LUNCH	DINNER
SUNDAY	Classic Eggs & Canadian Bacon	Traditional Falafel Pockets	Chopped Chicken–Brown Rice Salad
MONDAY	FAST	FAST	FAST
TUESDAY	Mixed Grain Porridge with Pear & Maple	Market Bulgur-Chicken Skillet	Pearl Barley–Turkey Soup
WEDNESDAY	FAST	FAST	FAST
THURSDAY	Creamy Mango-Jicama Smoothie	Pumpkin-Kale Tortilla Wraps	Salmon–Navy Bean Salad
FRIDAY	FAST	FAST	FAST
SATURDAY	Baked Egg & Herb Portobello Mushrooms	Pork Tenderloin Medallions with Herb Sauce	Cajun-Style Fish Tomato Stew

YOUR EXERCISE ROUTINE

Cardio workouts should be 30 minutes in duration, but you can work up to it if you are a beginner. Strength workouts should generally include three to four sets of 8 to 10 repetitions of each exercise where applicable. In the case of static core exercises, such as the plank, work toward holding the move longer each week.

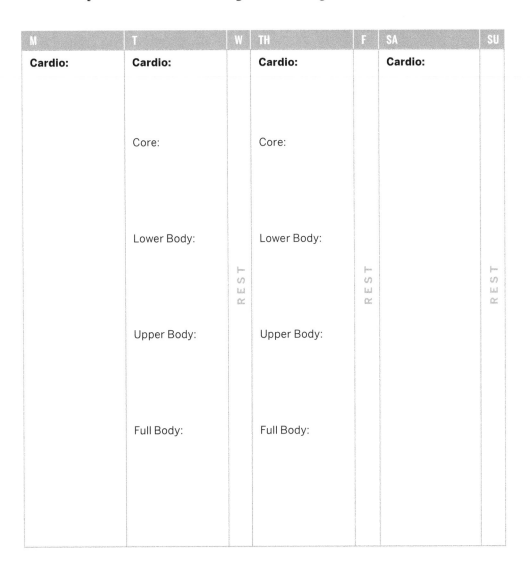

M	T	W	TH	F	SA	SU
Cardio:	**Cardio:**	REST	**Cardio:**	REST	**Cardio:**	REST
	Core:		Core:			
	Lower Body:		Lower Body:			
	Upper Body:		Upper Body:			
	Full Body:		Full Body:			

WELLNESS TRACKER

The wellness tracker is an optional but very useful tool to keep tabs on some of the important health behaviors that are encouraged in this book.

Your overall fasting duration, drinking enough water, sleeping eight hours a night, and eating multiple servings of fruits and vegetables are all very important habits you could choose to track using this helpful tool.

HABIT	M	T	W	TH	F	SA	SU
DRINK 8 GLASSES OF WATER	X		X			X	X

Week 3

I'm so thrilled to be welcoming you to week 3. While one leg of your intermittent fasting journey is about to end, I truly hope that this 21-day process only represents the beginning for you.

Whether you found a type of fasting you enjoy in week 1 or you are still getting there, hopefully by this point you've gained some appreciation of how flexible fasting can be. Even if you followed a relatively rigid structure up until this point, just know that beyond this final week you can play with fasting to make it work for you. The delicious recipes provided for week 3 will certainly help with that. Enjoy!

DAILY FASTS

Daily fasts, as usual, include 12:12, 16:8, and OMAD.

12:12

FASTING TIME	12 hours
EATING TIME	12 hours
CALORIES ALLOWED DURING FAST	None
MEALS PER DAY	3 meals per day, snacks optional

Congratulations on what is most likely your third week of 12:12 fasting. I hope it won't be your last!

Looking beyond these 21 days, I encourage you to adopt a flexible mind-set. You don't need to fast every day, nor do you need to fast for the same duration. If you want to skip fasting one day and go 14 hours the next, that's totally reasonable. Fasting should adapt to fit your life, not the other way around.

Remember you can feel free to replace any lunch recommendation with leftovers from dinner.

Congratulations again and enjoy week 3!

	BREAKFAST	**LUNCH**	**DINNER**
SUNDAY	Classic Eggs & Canadian Bacon	Curried Peanut Vegetable Noodles	Honey Sesame Salmon with Bok Choy
MONDAY	Fruit & Nut Yogurt Parfait	Fiery Pork Lettuce Wraps	Grain-&-Tofu-Stuffed Eggplant with Tahini
TUESDAY	Shrimp-Kale Omelet	Bulgur Lettuce Tacos	Chicken & Artichoke Heart Pita Pizzas
WEDNESDAY	Blueberry–Green Tea Smoothie	Chopped Chicken–Brown Rice Salad	Pan-Seared Trout with Dill & Leeks
THURSDAY	Baked Egg & Herb Portobello Mushrooms	Mediterranean Fish Tacos	Tofu Moussaka
FRIDAY	Mixed Grain Porridge with Pear & Maple	Edamame Mixed Green Salad with Berries	Pork–Bok Choy Chow Mein
SATURDAY	Ricotta-Oatmeal Pancakes	Pearl Barley–Turkey Soup	Baked Haddock-Mushroom Casserole

16:8

FASTING TIME	16 hours
EATING TIME	8 hours
CALORIES ALLOWED DURING FAST	None
MEALS PER DAY	2 meals per day, snacks optional *Note:* Beginners may choose to fast only on alternating days.

Welcome to week 3 of 16:8! This style of fast is an excellent choice moving forward after your first 21 days. Don't forget you have the option of slightly shortening (14:10) or extending (18:6) as your life and preferences dictate. Success with fasting in the long term will depend on embracing flexibility in your approach.

Remember you can replace any lunch recommendation with leftovers from dinner.

	BREAKFAST	LUNCH	DINNER
SUNDAY	FAST	North African–Inspired Shredded Vegetable Salad	Honey Sesame Salmon with Bok Choy
MONDAY	FAST	Fiery Pork Lettuce Wraps	Grain-&-Tofu-Stuffed Eggplant with Tahini
TUESDAY	FAST	Bulgur Lettuce Tacos	Chicken & Artichoke Heart Pita Pizzas
WEDNESDAY	FAST	Chopped Chicken–Brown Rice Salad	Pan-Seared Trout with Dill & Leeks
THURSDAY	FAST	Mediterranean Fish Tacos	Tofu Moussaka
FRIDAY	FAST	Edamame Mixed Green Salad with Berries	Pork–Bok Choy Chow Mein
SATURDAY	FAST	Pearl Barley–Turkey Soup	Baked Haddock-Mushroom Casserole

OMAD

FASTING TIME	22 to 23 hours
EATING TIME	1 to 2 hours
CALORIES ALLOWED DURING FAST	None
MEALS PER DAY	1 large meal per day *Note:* Remember to adjust the serving size for your one meal to reach your normal daily calories and add any supplemental snacks to ensure you are getting all your nutrients.

If you're on week 3 of OMAD, you've probably found it to be a great fit for you. I congratulate you and your progress so far. Ensure you are getting plenty of variety in your diet if you plan to continue OMAD beyond the first 21 days. If you are feeling adventurous and are new to OMAD in week 3, be sure to review the guidance provided in week 1.

	BREAKFAST	LUNCH	DINNER
SUNDAY	FAST	FAST	Honey Sesame Salmon with Bok Choy
MONDAY	FAST	FAST	Grain-&-Tofu-Stuffed Eggplant with Tahini
TUESDAY	FAST	FAST	Chicken & Artichoke Heart Pita Pizzas
WEDNESDAY	FAST	FAST	Pan-Seared Trout with Dill & Leeks
THURSDAY	FAST	FAST	Tofu Moussaka
FRIDAY	FAST	FAST	Pork–Bok Choy Chow Mein
SATURDAY	FAST	FAST	Baked Haddock-Mushroom Casserole

WEEKLY FASTS

Weekly fasts include 5:2, ADMF, and ADF.

5:2

FASTING DAYS PER WEEK	2
NORMAL EATING DAYS PER WEEK	5
CALORIES ALLOWED DURING FASTING DAYS	<800
MEALS PER DAY	All calories are eaten in within 1 to 8 hours on fasting days, either in one sitting on fasting days *or* two smaller meals.

Welcome to week 3 of 5:2 fasting! By now, I'm confident you know what it's all about. If you've been doing it since week 1, you may have landed on the style of fasting that will serve you for months and years to come.

If you are new to 5:2 fasting, be kind to yourself as you adapt to your fasted days. You may want to take it slow exercise-wise and allow yourself a bit more food if necessary. And remember that for days you are not fasting, feel free to replace any lunch recommendation with leftovers from dinner.

More details on 5:2 can be found in the week 1 section.

	BREAKFAST	LUNCH	DINNER
SUNDAY	Classic Eggs & Canadian Bacon	North African–Inspired Shredded Vegetable Salad	Honey Sesame Salmon with Bok Choy
MONDAY	FAST	Fiery Pork Lettuce Wraps	Grain-&-Tofu-Stuffed Eggplant with Tahini
TUESDAY	Shrimp-Kale Omelet	Bulgur Lettuce Tacos	Chicken & Artichoke Heart Pita Pizzas
WEDNESDAY	Blueberry–Green Tea Smoothie	Chopped Chicken–Brown Rice Salad	Pan-Seared Trout with Dill & Leeks
THURSDAY	FAST	Mediterranean Fish Tacos	Tofu Moussaka
FRIDAY	Mixed Grain Porridge with Pear & Maple	Edamame Mixed Green Salad with Berries	Pork–Bok Choy Chow Mein
SATURDAY	Ricotta-Oatmeal Pancakes	Pearl Barley–Turkey Soup	Baked Haddock-Mushroom Casserole

ALTERNATE-DAY MODIFIED

FASTING DAYS PER WEEK	3 to 4
NORMAL EATING DAYS PER WEEK	3 to 4
CALORIES ALLOWED DURING FAST	<800
MEALS PER DAY	All calories are eaten in within 1 to 8 hours on fasting days, either in one sitting on fasting days *or* two smaller meals. *Note:* Because alternating days can mean you either fast 3 or 4 days in a week, you can alter the difficulty of the fast by choosing whether the first day of the week is a fasting or eating day.

Welcome to week 3 of ADMF! I appreciate that going three days a week with a caloric limit can be challenging, so if you found it a bit too much, don't hesitate to consider trying 5:2 or allowing yourself 250 more calories on fasting days to make things more enjoyable. Don't forget to emphasize protein and fiber-rich meals, especially on fasting days.

If you are an experienced faster looking for a challenge beyond ADMF, alternate-day fasting is your best choice.

If you are new to ADMF this week, please refer to the detailed instructions in week 1.

Remember that for days you are not fasting, you can replace any lunch recommendation with leftovers from dinner.

	BREAKFAST	LUNCH	DINNER
SUNDAY	Classic Eggs & Canadian Bacon	North African–Inspired Shredded Vegetable Salad	Honey Sesame Salmon with Bok Choy
MONDAY	FAST	Fiery Pork Lettuce Wraps	Grain-&-Tofu-Stuffed Eggplant with Tahini
TUESDAY	Shrimp-Kale Omelet	Bulgur Lettuce Tacos	Chicken & Artichoke Heart Pita Pizzas
WEDNESDAY	FAST	Chopped Chicken–Brown Rice Salad	Pan-Seared Trout with Dill & Leeks
THURSDAY	Baked Egg & Herb Portobello Mushrooms	Mediterranean Fish Tacos	Tofu Moussaka
FRIDAY	FAST	Edamame Mixed Green Salad with Berries	Pork–Bok Choy Chow Mein
SATURDAY	Ricotta-Oatmeal Pancakes	Pearl Barley–Turkey Soup	Baked Haddock-Mushroom Casserole

FASTING DAYS PER WEEK	3 to 4 *Note:* Full day of fasting on alternating days
NORMAL EATING DAYS PER WEEK	3 to 4 *Note:* Full day of eating on alternating days
CALORIES ALLOWED DURING FAST	None
MEALS PER DAY	3 meals per day on eating days, snacks optional, none on fasting days *Note:* Because alternating days can mean you fast either 3 or 4 days in a week, you can alter the difficulty of the fast by choosing whether the first day of the week is a fasting or eating day.

If you are arriving at week 3 of alternate-day fasting and feel it's been a bit too much, don't forget you have other weekly fasts such as ADMF or 5:2 at your disposal.

If you enjoy alternate-day fasting and plan to continue, just be sure to be flexible in the sense that if you aren't up for a fasting day or want to break your fast because your body is demanding it, you should not feel bad doing so.

If you are new to alternate-day fasting in week 3, be sure to review the guidance offered in week 1.

Remember that for days you are not fasting, you are welcome to replace any lunch recommendation with leftovers from dinner.

	BREAKFAST	LUNCH	DINNER
SUNDAY	Classic Eggs & Canadian Bacon	North African–Inspired Shredded Vegetable Salad	Honey Sesame Salmon with Bok Choy
MONDAY	FAST	FAST	FAST
TUESDAY	Shrimp-Kale Omelet	Bulgur Lettuce Tacos	Chicken & Artichoke Heart Pita Pizzas
WEDNESDAY	FAST	FAST	FAST
THURSDAY	Baked Egg & Herb Portobello Mushrooms	Mediterranean Fish Tacos	Tofu Moussaka
FRIDAY	FAST	FAST	FAST
SATURDAY	Ricotta-Oatmeal Pancakes	Pearl Barley–Turkey Soup	Baked Haddock-Mushroom Casserole

YOUR EXERCISE ROUTINE

Cardio workouts should be 30 minutes in duration, but you can work up to it if you are a beginner. Strength workouts should generally include three to four sets of 8 to 10 repetitions of each exercise where applicable. In the case of static core exercises, such as the plank, work toward holding the move longer each week.

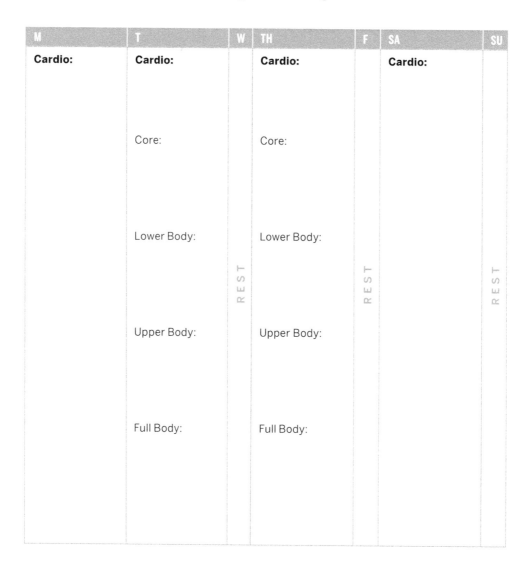

M	T	W	TH	F	SA	SU
Cardio:	**Cardio:**	REST	**Cardio:**	REST	**Cardio:**	REST
	Core:		Core:			
	Lower Body:		Lower Body:			
	Upper Body:		Upper Body:			
	Full Body:		Full Body:			

WELLNESS TRACKER

The wellness tracker is an optional but very useful tool to keep tabs on some of the important health behaviors that are encouraged in this book.

Your overall fasting duration, drinking enough water, sleeping eight hours a night, and eating multiple servings of fruits and vegetables are all very important habits you could choose to track using this helpful tool.

HABIT	M	T	W	TH	F	SA	SU
DRINK 8 GLASSES OF WATER	X		X			X	X

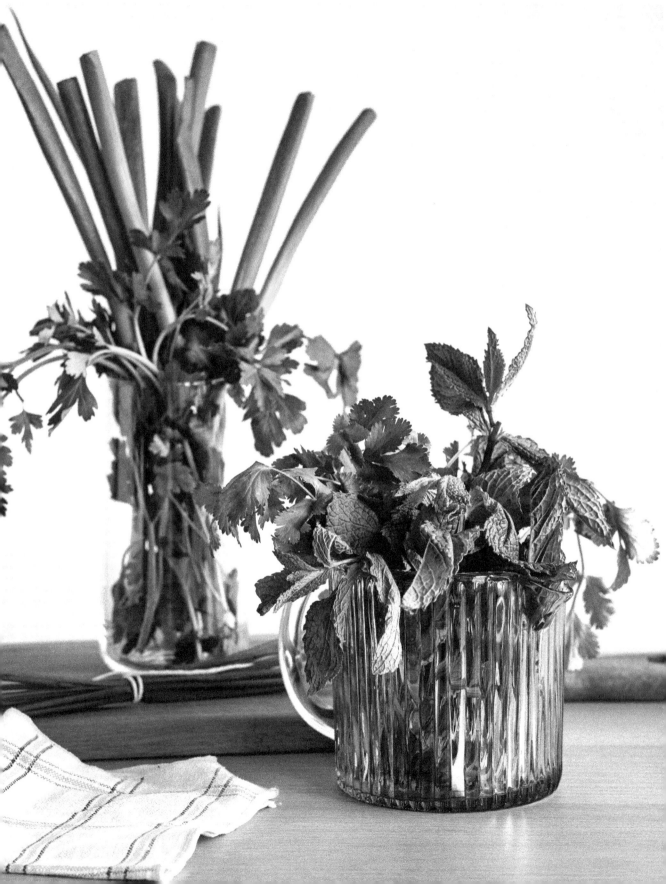

CHAPTER 4

TIPS FOR YOUR 21 DAYS—AND BEYOND

I'M HOPEFUL the first 21 days of your fasting journey will ultimately represent much more of a beginning than an end.

This chapter will provide you with additional insight to improve your chances of success in both the short and long term, while also discussing some of the science behind intermittent fasting and human health.

Breaking Your Fast

At its most fundamental level, intermittent fasting is about striking the perfect balance between what you give and what you get. This is true on the broader level, in the sense that you want to challenge yourself week-to-week and potentially try different types of fasts without ever feeling deprived or putting yourself through undue stress just for the sake of fasting a bit longer. It's also true on the day-to-day level. You should look forward to breaking your fast and knowing you will very likely enjoy the first post-fast meal a little bit more than usual. That's certainly one of the aspects I love most about it.

Intermittent fasting is not denying or starving yourself as some form of punishment. It is a very specific, dynamic strategy that takes advantage of biological and practical mechanisms to improve health. Admittedly, yes, it is something that requires getting used to.

You were provided a great deal of guidance in chapter 3 on when and how to break your fast. Some people may prefer a smaller first post-fast meal or even a snack before moving onto a larger meal. Others, such as those inclined to try OMAD, will be perfectly fine to eat one large meal and feel great doing so. There is no right or wrong answer here. A meal or snack that is healthy before fasting is still healthy after fasting, so listen to your body.

Where Fasting Can Benefit You

As scientists continue to explore the impact intermittent fasting could have on human health, I cannot help being both optimistic and excited about what the future holds. While the study of intermittent fasting is very much in its infancy, the early signs are more than encouraging.

Let's take a look at what the latest research has to say about the effects of fasting and some very important health concerns.

HIGH BLOOD PRESSURE

High blood pressure, also known as hypertension, is widely considered the number one preventable cause of death worldwide. It also happens to be one of the most common reasons why North Americans are prescribed medication by their doctors.

According to a 2019 paper in the journal *Nutrients*, intermittent fasting leads to increased production of a protein known as brain-derived neurotrophic factor, which stimulates brain cells to release the neurotransmitter acetylcholine. This chemical relaxes the heart and expands the vessels, contributing to lower blood pressure over time. Further, a 2018 study in the *Journal of the American Society of Hypertension* looked at intermittent fasting in people living with high blood pressure and found it had the potential to contribute to lower blood pressure throughout the day.

HIGH BLOOD CHOLESTEROL

Similar to high blood pressure, elevated blood cholesterol is a leading risk factor for death, disease, and doctor's visits across the United States.

There are very specific dietary steps a person can take to fight high cholesterol, with a plant-based diet being among the most effective.

Although intermittent fasting is not traditionally considered a treatment modality for elevated cholesterol, recent evidence from multiple studies suggests that perhaps it should be. A 2018 paper published by the European Society for Clinical Nutrition and Metabolism found evidence that fasting contributes to lower blood cholesterol levels but more research was required before definitive claims could be made. And in a 2018 *British Journal of Nutrition* paper, the researchers found that reducing caloric intake via intermittent fasting, rather than other methods, was more effective at lowering cholesterol levels.

INSULIN RESISTANCE AND TYPE 2 DIABETES

Insulin is an important hormone in blood sugar regulation because it stimulates your cells to take in the sugar from your blood for further processing. When your cells are not responding to insulin as they should, you develop a resistance to it, usually resulting in higher circulating blood sugar levels. Insulin resistance is a risk factor for type 2 diabetes, but it appears that intermittent fasting can help you fight back.

A 2018 study published in the journal *Cell Metabolism* looked at men living with prediabetes and found that, even without losing weight, intermittent fasting was shown to reduce insulin resistance. A 2011 study focusing on females in the *International Journal of Obesity* found that despite similarities in body fat loss between intermittent fasting and continuous energy restriction, there was evidence to suggest those engaged in fasting experienced greater reductions in insulin resistance. Although more research will certainly be necessary, these are the types of findings that get me excited about the potential role of intermittent fasting in the prevention of type 2 diabetes.

Cardiovascular disease is a leading—but largely preventable—killer of Americans and is driven at least in part by an inflammatory process known as atherosclerosis, the narrowing of arteries due to plaque buildup, which ultimately increases the risk of cardiovascular complications. A 2019 paper in *Nutrients* found that intermittent fasting reduced multiple inflammatory markers in the blood known to contribute to atherosclerotic plaque development.

Settling into Fasting Long-Term

As you continue your fasting journey beyond the 21-day plan, it's important to keep a few important points in mind to significantly improve your chances of success.

It all starts with having a bit of fun.

Make fasting fun. First and foremost: Enjoy the ride. I cannot stress enough how important it is that you really settle into a long-term routine that feels more like play than work. If you enjoy the process, you are more likely to keep at it.

Tailor it to fit your lifestyle. I've presented some strong evidence and arguments as to why fasting can offer you value, but experience is the best teacher. For the right person, the incorporation of intermittent fasting into their daily or weekly routine should simplify life, improve their health, and be genuinely low maintenance.

Although you've been presented specific 21-day plans in this book, intermittent fasting does not always need to be a strict, scheduled event. I certainly do not practice it that way. It is not a gimmick or quick-fix; rather, I see and use it as a dynamic tool based on simple principles that are meant to be used how you want to use them, when you want to use them. Want to fast one day? Do it. Don't want to fast the next? Don't.

For those who enjoy fasting, it will always be there for you. The real long-term joy of intermittent fasting is that you can fast when you want, for as long as you want, and you aren't ever forced to fast when you aren't up for it.

Don't be afraid to share your experience. I encourage you to share your fasting experience with those closest to you. After reading this book, you will surely have all sorts of fun facts and science to share with them—and given how popular intermittent fasting has become, they will probably be keen to hear what you have to say.

Important Fasting Considerations

Many people grow to truly enjoy intermittent fasting, but I also have to be honest in saying that fasting is not always fun and games. It comes with challenges that need to be considered, addressed, and managed.

LET'S TALK ABOUT HUNGER

Ah yes, the "H" word. *Hunger* is formally defined as the "compelling need or desire for food." Most people you ask would probably agree that their hunger tends to increase the further away they are from their last meal, depending on the context. The other thing many probably tend to agree on is the fact that they enjoy food more, and probably eat more, when they've gone an extended period of time without it. Anyone who has engaged in any sort of intermittent fasting will know exactly what I mean.

Here are some of my top tricks for combating hunger while fasting:

1. **Eat foods that are naturally satiating.** As part of your journey with intermittent fasting, you will inevitably test the limits of your hunger, and you should do so gradually while also focusing on eating healthy high-fiber, high-protein meals like the ones included in this book.

2. **Choose the style of fasting that's right for you.** Focusing on nutrient-dense and satiating meals will help, but so will discovering the style of fasting that is the best fit for you and your lifestyle. Put some serious thought into the information in chapters 2 and 3, and don't be afraid of some trial and error on your journey. Debilitating hunger is not the goal here; remember that fasting is meant to add to your quality of life, not detract from it, even if it may take some experimenting to arrive at that conclusion.

    The interaction between fasting and hunger is a fascinating one and is not as clear-cut as you might think. According to a 2015 review in the *Molecular and Cellular Endocrinology* journal, 10 different human trials looking at appetite and intermittent fasting found that appetite did not increase despite trial participants losing weight while fasting. Further evidence that intermittent fasting actually changes the way people experience hunger was demonstrated by a 2019 study in the journal *Obesity*. It looked at adults who carried out an 18:6 style of daily intermittent fasting over a four-day period where they ate only from 8 a.m. to 2 p.m. each day. As compared to those who ate the same number of calories over the full day, they found the intermittent fasters generally reported higher levels of fullness throughout the day, less hunger swings, and measurably lower levels of the hunger hormone ghrelin.

3. **Consider your circadian rhythm.** The style of fasting in the study described earlier, sometimes referred to as early time-restricted feeding (ETRF), may offer unique additional benefits because it is considered to be aligned with the human circadian rhythm. This is a biological internal clock in humans and mammals that helps regulate a wide variety of metabolic and physiological processes that at least partially depend on sleep/wake cycles associated with darkness, light, and the time of day. The manner in which your body functions, rests, and releases hormones varies throughout this 24-hour cycle. Insulin sensitivity decreases slightly throughout the day and into the night, which is why the ETRF style of fasting continues to garner extra attention. This may be an extra incentive for those intrigued by early time-restricted feeding.

4. **Enjoy fast-friendly broths and beverages.** Tea, black coffee, and good old-fashioned water can all be enjoyed while fasting. For something a little bit more interesting, broths and other fast-friendly beverage recipes can be found in chapter 10. Proper hydration, a little nutrient boost, and caffeine all play important roles in keeping you fueled, focused, and satisfied as you adapt to fasting.

SIDE EFFECTS AND DIETARY PATTERNS

All good things come with caveats and limitations, and intermittent fasting is no different. Keep in mind that intermittent fasting, great as it is, may not always be the right choice for you at every single point in time on any given day, week, or month. And that's okay. As I've mentioned, certain medications, life stages, and medical conditions simply may not align with fasting, especially the more extended styles. Having a super stressful or busy week may not be conducive to fasting, either. If you are unsure or have the slightest inclination to believe that fasting may run counter to the best interests of your health, consulting a health-care professional before proceeding is the wisest step.

There is one other essential topic to discuss before you embark on your journey into the world of intermittent fasting: the nutrient balance in your diet. My greatest concern about intermittent fasting in otherwise healthy people is that they miss out on certain important foods because they too strongly connect a time of day with eating a certain food.

Let's say, for example, you fall in love with a style of 16:8 intermittent fasting and end up rarely ever eating before noon. You've really enjoyed fasting and don't see yourself going back, but the meal you used to eat in the morning was pretty healthy. Let's say it was a yogurt parfait with nuts, seeds, and berries. Let's also assume that since you started fasting, you no longer eat that combination of foods because it's one you associate only with eating in the morning. As a dietitian, I see this pattern as particularly worrisome and not all that hard to fall into. The combination of foods in the yogurt parfait contains a number of unique nutritional benefits that are not easily or readily replicated in many other foods. Be aware of any omissions you may be making by eating at different times of the day. No one says, for example, that a yogurt parfait cannot be something you eat at noon, at 3 p.m., or even at 8 p.m.

It's important to think critically about your dietary patterns as you begin an intermittent fast, especially if you plan to pursue fasting in the long term.

Continuing Your Success

Thank you for joining me on this journey of exploration that has grown to become such a point of fascination in both my personal and professional lives. As research continues to emerge, I'm confident you will look back on your pursuit of fasting as being ahead of the curve. From the most basic benefits—simplifying your life and bringing variety to your days—to the more complex health benefits, like metabolic and biochemical impacts, there really is something to this concept of thinking about not just what you eat, but when you eat it.

Intermittent fasting, at the end of the day, is a dynamic tool meant to improve our quality of life. Implement and modify fasting as necessary to fit your life, and don't feel compelled to turn your life upside down to fit some predetermined fasting regimen. If you keep these points in mind, these same points I share with all of my clients who try it, I'm confident that both your enjoyment of the process and long-term success will be greatly improved.

So sit back, relax, and enjoy the ride.

PART II

RECIPES FOR YOUR FAST

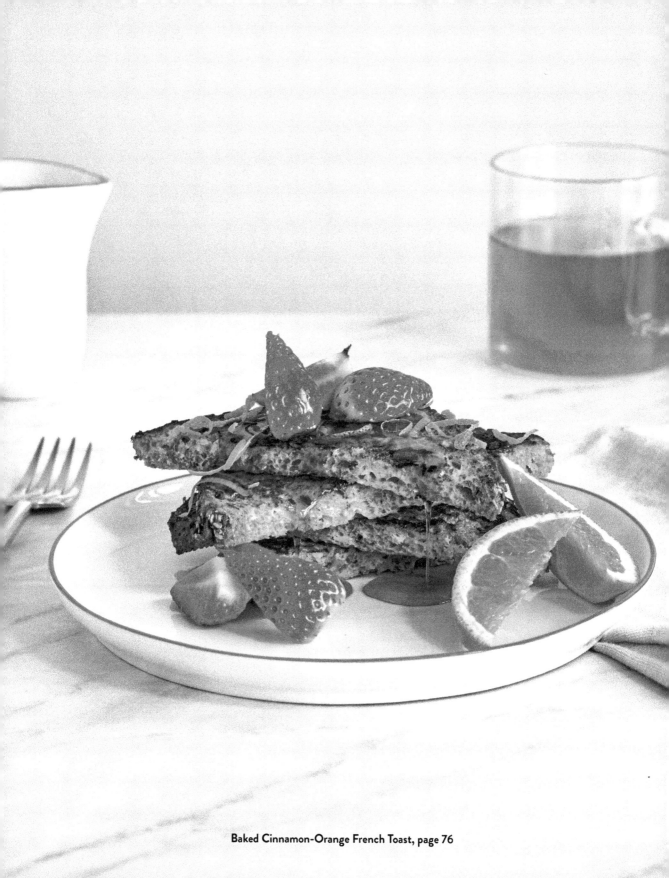

Baked Cinnamon-Orange French Toast, page 76

CHAPTER 5

BREAKFASTS & SMOOTHIES

Baked Cinnamon-Orange French Toast

SERVES 4 / PREP TIME: 10 MINUTES / COOK TIME: 12 MINUTES

30 MINUTES OR LESS, NUT-FREE, UNDER 500 CALORIES, VEGAN

French toast is a staple item on most restaurant brunch or breakfast menus because it is simple to make and absolutely delicious. This dish is thought to be of Roman origin and is a tasty way to use up stale bread. Baking the egg-drenched bread instead of frying the pieces in oil or butter cuts calories and fat considerably, creating a weight-loss-friendly meal.

Nonstick cooking spray
3 large eggs
½ cup skim milk or unsweetened almond milk
Juice and zest of 1 orange
¼ teaspoon ground cinnamon
8 slices multigrain bread
Maple syrup, for serving

1. Preheat the oven to 400°F.

2. Cover a baking sheet with parchment paper and lightly spray it with cooking spray. Set aside.

3. In a medium bowl, whisk together the eggs, milk, orange juice, orange zest, and cinnamon until well blended.

4. Lightly dredge each bread slice in the egg mixture and shake off any excess liquid.

5. Place the slices side by side on the baking sheet and very lightly spray the tops with cooking spray.

6. Bake until the bread is golden brown, then turn over each slice to brown, about 12 minutes.

7. Serve with a drizzle of maple syrup.

Addition Tip: Topping this delicious, filling breakfast with fresh berries or sliced banana will increase calories by about 100. Or if you add Rich Butter Coffee (page 155), calories increase to 440.

PER SERVING: Calories: 213; Total fat: 6g; Saturated fat: 2g; Sodium: 187mg; Carbohydrates: 27g; Fiber: 5g; Protein: 13g

Spicy Panzanella Breakfast Casserole

SERVES 4 / PREP TIME: 10 MINUTES / COOK TIME: 45 MINUTES

NUT-FREE, UNDER 500 CALORIES, VEGAN

Panzanella is an Italian salad that features tomatoes and bread cubes as well as other Mediterranean-inspired ingredients such as olives, peppers, onions, and cheese. Instead of tossing everything in a bowl with lettuce, you will be making a simple egg casserole. Fresh chopped basil is the ideal topping for this filling, protein-packed breakfast.

Nonstick cooking spray
2 cups cubed whole-grain bread
1 cup halved cherry tomatoes
1 teaspoon olive oil
1 yellow bell pepper, chopped
½ sweet onion, chopped
½ teaspoon minced garlic
6 large eggs, beaten
1 cup skim milk or unsweetened almond milk
Pinch red pepper flakes
Sea salt
Freshly ground black pepper
1 tablespoon chopped fresh basil

1. Preheat the oven to 325°F and use nonstick cooking spray to coat an 8-by-8-inch baking dish.

2. Arrange the bread cubes in the bottom of the baking dish and top them evenly with the tomatoes. Set aside.

3. Heat the oil in a medium skillet over medium-high heat.

4. Sauté the bell pepper, onion, and garlic until softened, about 4 minutes. Scatter the cooked vegetables over the bread and tomatoes.

5. In a small bowl, whisk together the eggs, milk, and red pepper flakes. Lightly season with salt and pepper.

6. Pour the egg mixture over the bread and vegetables.

7. Bake uncovered until the casserole is golden brown, 45 to 50 minutes.

8. Remove the casserole from the oven, and let it sit for 5 minutes before garnishing with basil and serving.

Make Ahead: You can put this dish together the night before, cover it, and bake it in the morning for 1 hour and 15 minutes.

PER SERVING: Calories: 233; Total fat: 10g; Saturated fat: 3g; Sodium: 273mg; Carbohydrates: 21g; Fiber: 3g; Protein: 16g

Mixed Grain Porridge with Pear & Maple

SERVES 4 / PREP TIME: 5 MINUTES / COOK TIME: 10 MINUTES

30 MINUTES OR LESS, ALLERGEN-FREE, DAIRY-FREE, NUT-FREE, ONE POT,
UNDER 500 CALORIES, VEGAN

Porridge is the ultimate comforting breakfast dish—nothing beats a thick steaming bowl of tender grains, fruit, and warm spices. Buckwheat might be an unusual choice for this recipe; its assertive flavor might be an acquired taste if you don't use this grain regularly. You can swap it out for more oats or quinoa, but buckwheat is packed with nutrients such as fiber and magnesium, so it's very good for the cardiovascular system and blood sugar levels.

½ cup rolled oats

¼ cup buckwheat

¼ cup quinoa, rinsed

1½ cups unsweetened vanilla almond milk, plus more for serving

1 cup water

1 cup diced pear

¼ teaspoon ground cinnamon

2 tablespoons maple syrup

½ cup roasted unsalted sunflower seeds, for garnish

1. Stir together the oats, buckwheat, quinoa, almond milk, water, pear, and cinnamon in a large saucepan, and place it over medium-high heat.

2. Bring the mixture to a boil, then reduce the heat to low, cover the saucepan, and simmer until the grains are tender and the liquid is almost all absorbed, about 10 minutes.

3. Remove from the heat and stir in the maple syrup.

4. Serve topped with sunflower seeds.

Craving Tip: The diced pear and drizzle of maple syrup will satisfy your craving for sweetness, while the grains and sunflower seeds provide filling fiber and healthy fats. If you are looking to eat more than 500 calories in one meal, double up the portion and enjoy!

PER SERVING: Calories: 269; Total fat: 12g; Saturated fat: 1g; Sodium: 138mg; Carbohydrates: 33g; Fiber: 7g; Protein: 9g

Ricotta-Oatmeal Pancakes

SERVES 4 / PREP TIME: 5 MINUTES / COOK TIME: 15 MINUTES

30 MINUTES OR LESS, UNDER 500 CALORIES, VEGAN

Oats are a stellar choice when following any fasting plan because this whole grain is high in filling fiber and protein. Oats are fat-free, low-calorie, and high in calcium and iron. Including oats regularly in your diet can reduce your risk of heart disease and cancer, as well as stabilize blood sugar and decrease blood pressure.

2 large eggs
½ cup ricotta cheese
1 tablespoon honey
1 tablespoon melted coconut oil
1 teaspoon pure vanilla extract
½ cup rolled oats
¼ cup almond flour
1 teaspoon baking powder
¼ teaspoon ground nutmeg
Nonstick cooking spray
½ cup maple syrup

1. Place the eggs, ricotta cheese, honey, oil, and vanilla in a blender and pulse 30 seconds.

2. Add the oats, almond flour, baking powder, and nutmeg to the blender and pulse until well blended, about 30 seconds.

3. Place a large skillet over medium heat, and lightly coat it with cooking spray.

4. Pour about a quarter cup of batter onto the skillet for each pancake, about four per batch; do not overcrowd.

5. Cook until the tops of the pancakes start to bubble, about 3 minutes, then flip the pancakes over.

6. Cook until the pancakes are completely cooked through and golden brown on both sides, about 2 minutes more.

7. Repeat with the remaining batter.

8. Serve warm or cold with maple syrup.

Make Ahead: Store these tender pancakes in the refrigerator, individually wrapped with pieces of parchment. Try them cold, wrapped around fresh fruit, for a quick grab-and-go meal.

PER SERVING: Calories: 284; Total fat: 11g; Saturated fat: 5g; Sodium: 55mg; Carbohydrates: 40g; Fiber: 3g; Protein: 7g

Shrimp-Kale Omelet

SERVES 3 / PREP TIME: 10 MINUTES / COOK TIME: 8 MINUTES

30 MINUTES OR LESS, NUT-FREE, UNDER 500 CALORIES

This omelet is absolutely lovely, and the earthy flavor of the kale is perfectly balanced by tender, sweet chunks of shrimp. Shrimp is an excellent source of protein in a low-calorie package—a dozen shrimp are less than 100 calories. This shellfish is also high in B12, iron, selenium, and vitamin D, so it can help reduce inflammation in the body and boost the immune system.

6 large eggs
½ teaspoon chopped fresh dill
Sea salt
Freshly ground black pepper
1 tablespoon butter
1 tablespoon olive oil
1 cup chopped fresh baby kale
2 tablespoons chopped sweet onion
1 cup chopped cooked shrimp
½ cup halved cherry tomatoes

1. In a small bowl, whisk together the eggs and dill, and lightly season with salt and pepper. Set aside.

2. Melt the butter in a large skillet over medium-high heat and add the oil.

3. Sauté the kale and onion until the greens are wilted, about 3 minutes.

4. Pour the egg mixture into the skillet, and cook until barely set, about 4 minutes, lifting the edges to allow the uncooked egg to pour underneath.

5. When the eggs are set, scatter the shrimp and tomatoes evenly over the top.

6. Fold the omelet over to create a half-moon and allow to cook for 1 minute more.

7. Cut the omelet into thirds and serve immediately.

Variation Tip: Cooked chicken would also make a nice addition to this omelet. Eight ounces of chicken breast would add 60 calories and 10 grams of protein per serving.

PER SERVING: Calories: 304; Total fat: 19g; Saturated fat: 7g; Sodium: 312mg; Carbohydrates: 6g; Fiber: 1g; Protein: 27g

Avocado, Roasted Red Pepper & Tofu Scramble

SERVES 4 / PREP TIME: 10 MINUTES / COOK TIME: 12 MINUTES

30 MINUTES OR LESS, DAIRY-FREE, NUT-FREE, UNDER 500 CALORIES, VEGAN

You might be wondering if adding avocado to the other ingredients creates a green scramble à la Dr. Seuss. It does not, but the scramble is still very attractive, with bits of deep red pepper, dark green herbs, pastel avocado chunks, and pale yellow fluffy eggs. Make sure the avocado is ripe but not mushy to create the perfect texture. If the fruit is a bit too firm, place it overnight in a paper bag with a ripe banana; the ethylene gas the banana gives off can help the avocado ripen quicker.

6 large eggs

1 teaspoon chopped fresh basil

1 teaspoon chopped fresh oregano

1 tablespoon olive oil

¼ cup chopped sweet onion

½ teaspoon minced garlic

1 cup diced extra-firm tofu

1 cup chopped jarred roasted red pepper

1 avocado, pitted, peeled and diced

1 tablespoon chopped fresh parsley

Sea salt

Freshly ground black pepper

1. In a small bowl, whisk together the eggs, basil, and oregano and set aside.

2. Heat the oil in a large skillet over medium-high heat.

3. Sauté the onion and garlic until softened, about 3 minutes.

4. Add the tofu and red pepper to the skillet, and sauté until the tofu is heated through, about 6 minutes.

5. Pour the egg mixture into the skillet, and scramble until fluffy curds form and the eggs are just cooked through but still shiny, about 3 minutes.

6. Remove the skillet from the heat, and fold in the avocado and parsley.

7. Season with salt and pepper and serve immediately.

Addition Tip: Wrap this savory mixture in a large multigrain tortilla or stuff into pita bread. This will add about 200 calories per serving, creating a meal more than 500 calories.

PER SERVING: Calories: 307; Total fat: 19g; Saturated fat: 4g; Sodium: 310mg; Carbohydrates: 13g; Fiber: 4g; Protein: 18g

Date-Fennel Smoothie

SERVES 2 / PREP TIME: 8 MINUTES

Fennel is a member of the same family as parsley, carrots, and dill and is topped with similar edible feathery fronds. Fennel adds fiber and phytonutrients to this beverage, and an appealing licorice-like flavor to the sweet dates and pear. Fennel can reduce cholesterol, stabilize blood sugar, and fight disease-causing inflammation.

1 pear, cored
4 Medjool dates
2 cups fresh baby spinach
1 cup chopped fennel
½ cup unsweetened apple juice
2 tablespoons hemp hearts
Pinch ground nutmeg
4 ice cubes

1. Place the pear, dates, spinach, fennel, apple juice, hemp hearts, and nutmeg in a blender and pulse until smooth.

2. Add the ice cubes and blend until the drink is smooth.

3. Pour the smoothie into two glasses and serve immediately.

Addition Tip: Add a couple of scoops of vanilla or unflavored protein powder to the smoothie to increase the calories by about 100 and the protein by 20 to 22 grams per serving.

PER SERVING: Calories: 319; Total fat: 7g; Saturated fat: 1g; Sodium: 61mg; Carbohydrates: 60g; Fiber: 9g; Protein: 9g

Almond Butter–Quinoa Smoothie

SERVES 2 / PREP TIME: 5 MINUTES

30 MINUTES OR LESS, ONE POT, UNDER 500 CALORIES, VEGAN

Apples aren't the main ingredient in this rich protein- and fiber-packed smoothie, but they do add essential nutrients and a subtly sweet flavor. Apples are a fabulous source of fiber, vitamins C and B, calcium, and antioxidants. Eating an apple a day can cut the risk of most chronic diseases, such as diabetes, cancer, and cardiovascular disease.

1 apple, peeled, cored, and grated
½ cup cooked quinoa
½ cup vanilla Greek yogurt
½ cup unsweetened almond milk
2 tablespoons almond butter
Pinch ground cinnamon
2 cups ice cubes

1. Place the apple, quinoa, yogurt, almond milk, almond butter, and cinnamon in a blender and pulse until smooth.

2. Add the ice cubes and blend until smooth.

3. Pour into two glasses and serve immediately.

Make Ahead: Cook the quinoa ahead using a 1:2 ratio of quinoa to water. Bring the mixture to a boil, reduce the heat to low, cover, and simmer for 15 minutes until the liquid is absorbed.

PER SERVING: Calories: 334; Total fat: 13g; Saturated fat: 1g; Sodium: 69mg; Carbohydrates: 46g; Fiber: 7g; Protein: 12g

Blueberry–Green Tea Smoothie

SERVES 2 / PREP TIME: 5 MINUTES, PLUS CHILL TIME / COOK TIME: 5 MINUTES

30 MINUTES OR LESS, NUT-FREE, UNDER 500 CALORIES

Blueberries add a pretty color and complex sweetness to this smoothie, offsetting the tart kefir and slightly bitter kale. Blueberries are fiber-rich and low on the glycemic index, perfect for creating a feeling of fullness without unpleasant blood sugar spikes. Of all fruits and vegetables, blueberries have one of the highest antioxidant levels, so they can protect against disease and aging.

2 cups boiling water
2 green tea bags
2 cups fresh blueberries
2 cups unsweetened vanilla kefir
1 cup baby kale
1 scoop vanilla protein powder
2 tablespoons honey
3 ice cubes

1. Place the water in a liquid measuring cup, add the tea bags, and steep for about 5 minutes, then remove the tea bags.

2. Place the tea in the refrigerator until cool, about 20 minutes.

3. Place the tea, blueberries, kefir, kale, protein powder, and honey in a blender and pulse until smooth.

4. Add the ice cubes and blend until the drink is smooth.

5. Pour into two glasses and serve immediately.

Make Ahead: Brew the tea and cool in the refrigerator until you wish to make the smoothie. You can even make the tea the evening before if this beverage is for breakfast.

PER SERVING: Calories: 358; Total fat: 7g; Saturated fat: 3g; Sodium: 159mg; Carbohydrates: 54g; Fiber: 4g; Protein: 23g

Creamy Mango-Jicama Smoothie

SERVES 2 / PREP TIME: 5 MINUTES

30 MINUTES OR LESS, NUT-FREE, ONE POT, UNDER 500 CALORIES

Mango and jicama might seem like an unusual combination, but the pairing creates a filling, delicious beverage ideal for a quick meal. Mango is high in amino acids, beta-carotene, calcium, and vitamin C, and jicama is packed with fiber, B vitamins, vitamin A, and iron. This mixture of nutrients stabilizes blood sugar, supports healthy digestion, and cuts the risk of diabetes, cancer, and anemia.

1 mango, peeled, pitted, and cut into chunks
1 cup shredded jicama
2 cups plain Greek yogurt
1 scoop vanilla protein powder
1 teaspoon pure vanilla extract
Pinch ground cinnamon
3 cups ice cubes

1. Place the mango, jicama, yogurt, protein powder, vanilla, and cinnamon in a blender and pulse until smooth.

2. Add the ice cubes and blend until smooth.

3. Pour into glasses and serve immediately.

Variation Tip: If you can't find jicama, you can throw in fennel or parsnip instead. Just shred the vegetable and add 1 cup to this exotic smoothie. The change won't significantly affect the calories.

PER SERVING: Calories: 372; Total fat: 2g; Saturated fat: 1g; Sodium: 168mg; Carbohydrates: 46g; Fiber: 6g; Protein: 45g

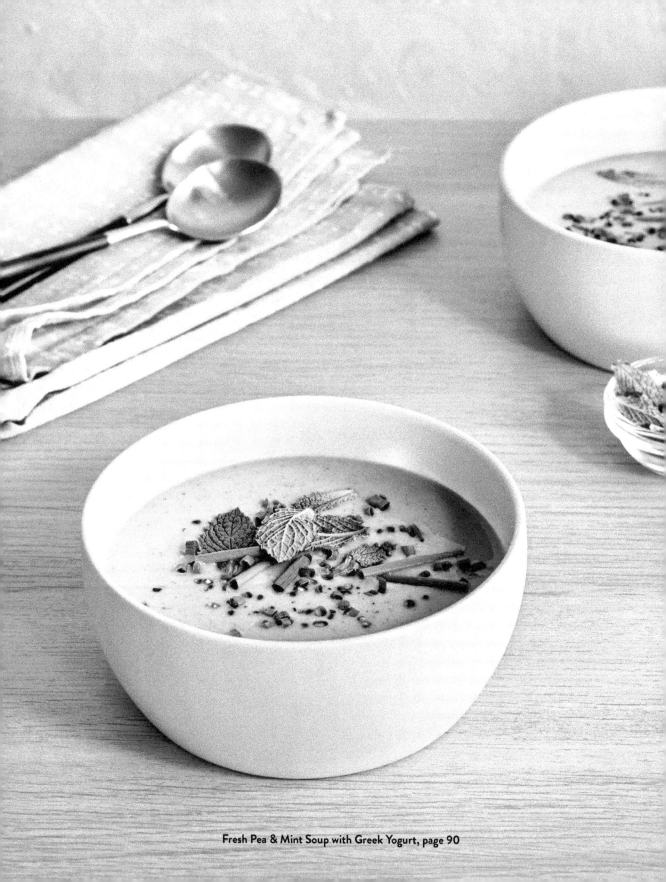

Fresh Pea & Mint Soup with Greek Yogurt, page 90

CHAPTER 6

SOUPS & SALADS

Bistro Tomato Soup with Kefir Drizzle

SERVES 4 / PREP TIME: 15 MINUTES / COOK TIME: 30 MINUTES

NUT-FREE, UNDER 500 CALORIES, VEGAN

Tomato soup can get a bad reputation because canned products are often watery and pale. Real homemade tomato soup is a glorious deep red color and bursting with the flavor of summer. Tomatoes are an excellent source of vitamins A, C, and K, as well as fiber. This fruit also contains a disease-fighting phytonutrient called lycopene that becomes more bioavailable when heated up, so enjoy this soup warm.

1 tablespoon olive oil

1 sweet onion,
   finely chopped

2 celery stalks, chopped

1 carrot, shredded

1 tablespoon
   minced garlic

2 (28-ounce) cans
   low-sodium diced
   tomatoes

4 cups low-sodium
   vegetable broth

2 tablespoons chopped
   fresh basil

1 teaspoon chopped
   fresh oregano

Sea salt

Freshly ground
   black pepper

1 cup plain kefir

1. Heat the oil in a large pot on medium-high heat.

2. Sauté the onion, celery, carrot, and garlic until softened, about 5 minutes.

3. Stir in the tomatoes and broth and bring the soup to a boil.

4. Reduce the heat to low and simmer the soup until the vegetables are tender, about 25 minutes.

5. Remove the soup from the heat, and purée with an immersion blender or in a food processor until almost smooth. A little texture is delicious.

6. Transfer the soup back to the saucepan and stir in the basil and oregano.

7. Season with salt and pepper and serve with a generous drizzle of kefir.

Make Ahead: This soup freezes very well, so double the recipe, cool, and package into 1-cup serving containers. Label with the date and freeze for up to 3 months. Do not add the kefir until the soup is reheated, because this ingredient should not be frozen.

PER SERVING: Calories: 201; Total fat: 5g; Saturated fat: 1g; Sodium: 198mg; Carbohydrates: 30g; Fiber: 6g; Protein: 8g

Sweet Potato–Orange Soup

SERVES 4 / PREP TIME: 15 MINUTES / COOK TIME: 35 MINUTES

ALLERGEN-FREE, DAIRY-FREE, NUT-FREE, UNDER 500 CALORIES

Soups can be the ideal method to warm you up on chilly fall and winter days, especially when those soups are composed of autumn vegetables and warm spices. Sweet potato and orange create a palate-pleasing combination that would be even better with a swirl of yogurt or sour cream, which would add protein and vitamin B6 and help support a healthy cardiovascular system.

1 tablespoon olive oil

**1 sweet onion,
   finely chopped**

**1 tablespoon peeled
   grated fresh ginger**

2 teaspoons minced garlic

**5 cups low-sodium
   chicken broth**

**4 sweet potatoes, peeled
   and diced**

Juice and zest of 1 orange

1 tablespoon maple syrup

**1 teaspoon
   ground nutmeg**

**¼ teaspoon ground
   cinnamon**

Sea salt

**Freshly ground
   black pepper**

1. Heat the oil in a large stockpot over medium-high heat.

2. Sauté the onion, ginger, and garlic until softened, about 4 minutes.

3. Stir in the broth, sweet potatoes, orange juice and zest, maple syrup, nutmeg, and cinnamon.

4. Bring the soup to a boil, then reduce the heat to low and simmer until the vegetables are tender, 25 to 30 minutes.

5. Remove the soup from the heat, and purée with a blender or immersion blender until smooth.

6. Season to taste with salt and pepper and serve.

Addition Tip: Serve this lovely soup with a salad such as the Kale Salad with Peach & Blue Cheese (page 92) to increase calories to 500 per serving. The combination of earthy greens and sweet soup is stellar.

PER SERVING: Calories: 210; Total fat: 4g; Saturated fat: 1g; Sodium: 151mg; Carbohydrates: 37g; Fiber: 5g; Protein: 7g

Fresh Pea & Mint Soup with Greek Yogurt

SERVES 4 / PREP TIME: 10 MINUTES / COOK TIME: 5 MINUTES

30 MINUTES OR LESS, NUT-FREE, UNDER 500 CALORIES, VEGAN

Peas and mint are a classic spring combination because both ingredients are bright and fresh in spring. You can certainly make this splendid soup any season if using flash-frozen peas, but it is best with just-picked produce. The Greek yogurt mellows the color a little and adds about 10 grams of protein to this high-fiber meal. You can also use sour cream or kefir for a similar flavor.

1 tablespoon olive oil

½ cup chopped sweet onion

4 cups low-sodium vegetable broth

6 cups fresh or frozen green peas

¼ cup fresh chopped mint

½ cup plain Greek yogurt

Sea salt

Freshly ground black pepper

1 tablespoon chopped fresh chives, for garnish

1. Heat the oil in a large saucepan over medium-high heat.

2. Sauté the onion until softened, about 3 minutes.

3. Stir in the broth and bring to a boil.

4. Stir in the peas and cook for 2 to 3 minutes, until the peas are tender.

5. Remove from the heat and stir in the mint.

6. Purée the soup in a blender until very smooth.

7. Transfer the soup back to the saucepan and whisk in the yogurt.

8. Season with salt and pepper and serve topped with chives.

Craving Tip: This soup is not packed with calories, but it has such an incredibly fresh taste you will feel satisfied after a bowl, especially if you add a tablespoon of honey with the yogurt to enhance its natural sweetness.

PER SERVING: Calories: 240; Total fat: 4g; Saturated fat: 1g; Sodium: 161mg; Carbohydrates: 36g; Fiber: 12g; Protein: 14g

Creamy Vegetable-Tofu Soup

SERVES 4 / PREP TIME: 20 MINUTES / COOK TIME: 30 MINUTES

DAIRY-FREE, NUT-FREE, UNDER 500 CALORIES, VEGAN

Onions are a common ingredient in most savory recipes; added along with other vegetables, they create a pleasing flavor. Onions are more than an assumed recipe addition; they are also very rich in flavonoids such as quercetin. Quercetin supports the cardiovascular system and can reduce the risk of cancer and diabetes. You can also use leeks or shallots in this recipe with similar effects and flavor.

1 tablespoon olive oil

1 sweet onion, chopped

2 celery stalks, chopped

1 tablespoon minced garlic

6 cups low-sodium vegetable broth

8 ounces silken tofu

2 cups chopped cauliflower

2 parsnips, chopped

2 carrots, chopped

1 cup low-sodium canned navy beans, drained and rinsed

1 cup shredded fresh baby spinach

Sea salt

Freshly ground black pepper

1. Heat the oil in a large pot over medium-high heat.

2. Sauté the onion, celery, and garlic until softened, about 5 minutes.

3. Add the broth and bring to a boil.

4. Stir in the tofu, cauliflower, parsnips, carrots, and navy beans and reduce the heat to low.

5. Cover the saucepan and simmer until the vegetables are tender, about 25 minutes.

6. Transfer the soup to a food processor and purée until smooth.

7. Transfer the soup back to the saucepan and stir in the spinach.

8. Season with salt and pepper and serve.

Addition Tip: If you want to add more protein to the soup, increase the tofu to 16 ounces. This will add 4 to 5 grams of protein per serving, which helps you feel full longer when combined with high-quality carbs.

PER SERVING: Calories: 243; Total fat: 6g; Saturated fat: 1g; Sodium: 152mg; Carbohydrates: 36g; Fiber: 11g; Protein: 15g

Kale Salad with Peach & Blue Cheese

SERVES 4 / PREP TIME: 5 MINUTES

30 MINUTES OR LESS, NUT-FREE, ONE POT, UNDER 500 CALORIES, VEGAN

Kale is considered a superfood because of its incredible array of nutrients, but it can also be a bit hard to eat or digest depending on the particular bunch and how often you consume it. Mature kale leaves are actually quite woody and have a hard texture because of the fiber content, so it can cause upper stomach bloating and indigestion. If you have not eaten a great deal of kale, ease into it slowly by using half kale and half regular lettuce in this recipe, and make sure the kale you purchase is tender baby greens.

8 cups baby kale

¼ cup Oil & Vinegar Dressing (page 170)

2 cups halved cherry tomatoes

2 peaches, pitted and thinly sliced

1 scallion, white and green parts, thinly sliced on a bias

½ cup crumbled blue cheese

¼ cup roasted unsalted pumpkin seeds

1. In a large bowl, toss the kale with the dressing to coat the greens.

2. Add the tomatoes, peaches, and scallion and toss to mix.

3. Arrange the salads on four plates, and evenly divide the blue cheese and pumpkin seeds among them before serving.

Addition Tip: Include a 5-ounce grilled or baked chicken breast with each portion of salad to increase the calories by 185 and the protein by 34 grams per serving.

PER SERVING: Calories: 291; Total fat: 16g; Saturated fat: 5g; Sodium: 276mg; Carbohydrates: 27g; Fiber: 5g; Protein: 12g

Pearl Barley–Turkey Soup

SERVES 4 / PREP TIME: 20 MINUTES / COOK TIME: 30 MINUTES

ALLERGEN-FREE, DAIRY-FREE, NUT-FREE, ONE POT, UNDER 500 CALORIES

Beef barley soup is probably the version of this dish you have seen over the years, but turkey is just as tasty and nutritious as beef. This is the ideal recipe for leftover turkey from holiday meals. Barley is one of those grains that might not be a regular choice in your meals, but it should be because it is exceptionally high in niacin and fiber, both insoluble and soluble. Barley can lower cholesterol and reduce the risk of atherosclerosis.

1 tablespoon olive oil
1 sweet onion, chopped
3 celery stalks, chopped
1 tablespoon
   minced garlic
6 cups low-sodium
   chicken broth
½ cup pearl barley
2 carrots, diced
1 sweet potato, diced
1 bay leaf
2 cups chopped
   cooked turkey
1 cup fresh green beans,
   cut into 1-inch pieces
Sea salt
Freshly ground
   black pepper
1 tablespoon chopped
   fresh parsley,
   for garnish

1. Heat the oil in a large saucepan over medium-high heat.

2. Sauté the onion, celery, and garlic until softened, about 5 minutes.

3. Add the broth, barley, carrots, sweet potato, and bay leaf.

4. Bring the soup to a boil, then reduce the heat to medium-low and simmer until the barley and vegetables are tender, about 20 minutes.

5. Remove the bay leaf and stir in the turkey and green beans.

6. Simmer 5 minutes more to heat through.

7. Season with salt and pepper and serve topped with parsley.

Variation Tip: Wild rice, bulgur, lentils, or navy beans can take the place of the barley in this filling, rustic soup. If you use canned beans, the cooking time will not increase.

PER SERVING: Calories: 325; Total fat: 7g; Saturated fat: 2g; Sodium: 187mg; Carbohydrates: 35g; Fiber: 7g; Protein: 28g

Edamame Mixed Green Salad with Berries

SERVES 4 / PREP TIME: 25 MINUTES

30 MINUTES OR LESS, ONE POT, UNDER 500 CALORIES, VEGAN

Edamame is immature soybeans still in an inedible pod, although you can buy them shelled for convenience. This ingredient adds a different texture and shape to the chopped and shredded salad, as well as about 10 grams of protein per serving. When combined with fiber-rich broccoli and asparagus, you get a fabulous meal for a fasting diet. Asparagus and broccoli are high in antioxidants, can detox the body, and can reduce the risk of cancer and cardiovascular disease.

4 cups mixed greens

2 cups chopped broccoli

1 cup shredded asparagus

2 cups edamame

2 cups mixed fresh berries (strawberries, blueberries, raspberries, blackberries)

½ cup Honeyed Buttermilk Dressing (page 163)

½ cup chopped pecans

1. In a large bowl, toss together the mixed greens, broccoli, asparagus, and edamame.

2. Arrange the salads on four plates, and evenly divide the berries among them.

3. Drizzle the salads with the dressing and top with pecans before serving.

Variation Tip: Kale, spinach, or Swiss chard can take the place of standard mixed greens. Choose baby greens or chop mature kale and spinach into bite-size pieces before adding to the salad.

PER SERVING: Calories: 328; Total fat: 15g; Saturated fat: 2g; Sodium: 135mg; Carbohydrates: 35g; Fiber: 11g; Protein: 20g

Chopped Chicken–Brown Rice Salad

SERVES 4 / PREP TIME: 25 MINUTES

30 MINUTES OR LESS, DAIRY-FREE, ONE POT, UNDER 500 CALORIES

Brown rice is a crucial ingredient in many fasting plans going back thousands of years; folks supposedly cleansed and detoxed the body by eating nothing other than 3 to 6 cups of brown rice per day. Brown rice is thought to be grounding and warming in both macrobiotic and Ayurvedic traditions. This grain is very high in iron, magnesium, and B vitamins, so it can provide energy if this tasty salad is your meal for the day.

2 cups cooked brown rice

1 cup cooked low-sodium lentils

1 cup chopped cooked chicken breasts

1 cup snow peas, cut into ½-inch pieces

1 cup shredded carrot

1 red bell pepper, diced

1 scallion, white and green parts, thinly sliced

¼ cup Orange-Cilantro Vinaigrette (page 169)

¼ cup chopped pistachios

1. In a large bowl, toss together the brown rice, lentils, chicken, snow peas, carrot, bell pepper, and scallion until well mixed.

2. Add the dressing and toss to combine.

3. Serve topped with pistachios.

Make Ahead: Soaking brown rice will cut the cooking time. Place 2 cups of rice in a bowl with 4 cups of warm water and let it sit at room temperature for at least 2 hours or overnight. Drain and add 3 cups of water and bring to a boil over high heat. Reduce the heat to low, cover, and simmer until the liquid is absorbed, about 20 minutes.

PER SERVING: Calories: 331; Total fat: 13g; Saturated fat: 2g; Sodium: 81mg; Carbohydrates: 35g; Fiber: 7g; Protein: 19g

North African-Inspired Shredded Vegetable Salad

SERVES 4 / PREP TIME: 10 MINUTES, PLUS 2 HOURS CHILL TIME

DAIRY-FREE, ONE POT, UNDER 500 CALORIES, VEGAN

Many of the vegetables in this delightful salad are not traditional to North African cuisine, but the spices and flavors make up for this deviation. Red cabbage adds impressive color and a hefty portion of vitamins C and K, plus fiber to the dish. Red cabbage is also high in phytonutrients such as anthocyanin, which creates the vibrant deep color of this vegetable and protects against heart disease and cancer. Cabbage comes in a range of colors from deep, dark red to a bright purple. The color is dependent on the pH in the soil: redder for acidic soils, and purple for neutral soils.

¼ cup olive oil

2 tablespoons apple cider vinegar

Juice of 1 lemon

1 tablespoon honey

1 tablespoon chopped fresh parsley

1 teaspoon minced garlic

½ teaspoon ground cumin

¼ teaspoon ground coriander

4 cups shredded carrot

2 cups shredded parsnip

1 cup shredded red cabbage

1 cup shredded jicama

1 apple, cored and shredded

½ cup chopped almonds

1. In a large bowl, whisk together the oil, vinegar, lemon juice, honey, parsley, garlic, cumin, and coriander.

2. Add the carrot, parsnip, cabbage, jicama, apple, and almonds.

3. Toss to coat the vegetables and place the salad in the refrigerator for 2 hours to let the spices mellow before serving.

Make Ahead: This salad is even better the second day when the spices have mellowed, so throw it together the day before you wish to serve it or double the recipe to create tasty leftovers. The lemon in the salad will prevent the apple from oxidizing as the dish sits in your refrigerator.

PER SERVING: Calories: 339; Total fat: 19g; Saturated fat: 2g; Sodium: 91mg; Carbohydrates: 41g; Fiber: 11g; Protein: 7g

Salmon–Navy Bean Salad

SERVES 4 / PREP TIME: 20 MINUTES

30 MINUTES OR LESS, ALLERGEN-FREE, DAIRY-FREE, NUT-FREE, ONE POT,
UNDER 500 CALORIES

Salmon is one of those versatile ingredients that can be enjoyed either fresh or canned, depending on availability and your budget. It is very high in protein and heart-friendly omega-3 fatty acids. Whenever possible, try to find wild-caught fish because it is lower in saturated fat and sodium and higher in potassium, calcium, and zinc. If you want a single meal of about 700 calories, double this recipe and enjoy!

¼ cup olive oil

1 tablespoon apple
  cider vinegar

Juice and zest of 1 lemon

1 (15-ounce) can
  low-sodium navy beans,
  drained and rinsed

3 cups chopped baby kale

1 English cucumber, diced

1 yellow bell pepper, diced

4 radishes, sliced

Sea salt

Freshly ground
  black pepper

2 (6.5-ounces) cans
  low-sodium
  water-packed
  salmon, drained

1 tablespoon chopped
  fresh parsley

1. In a large bowl, whisk together the oil, vinegar, and lemon juice and zest.

2. Add the navy beans, kale, cucumber, bell pepper, and radishes to the bowl and toss to coat.

3. Season the salad with salt and pepper.

4. Top with the salmon and parsley and serve.

Variation Tip: Water-packed canned tuna or left-over baked fish can be used instead of salmon in this pretty salad. The protein and calories will be similar, and the fat grams will decrease slightly.

PER SERVING: Calories: 359; Total fat: 14g;
Saturated fat: 2g; Sodium: 312mg; Carbohydrates: 29g;
Fiber: 10g; Protein: 26g

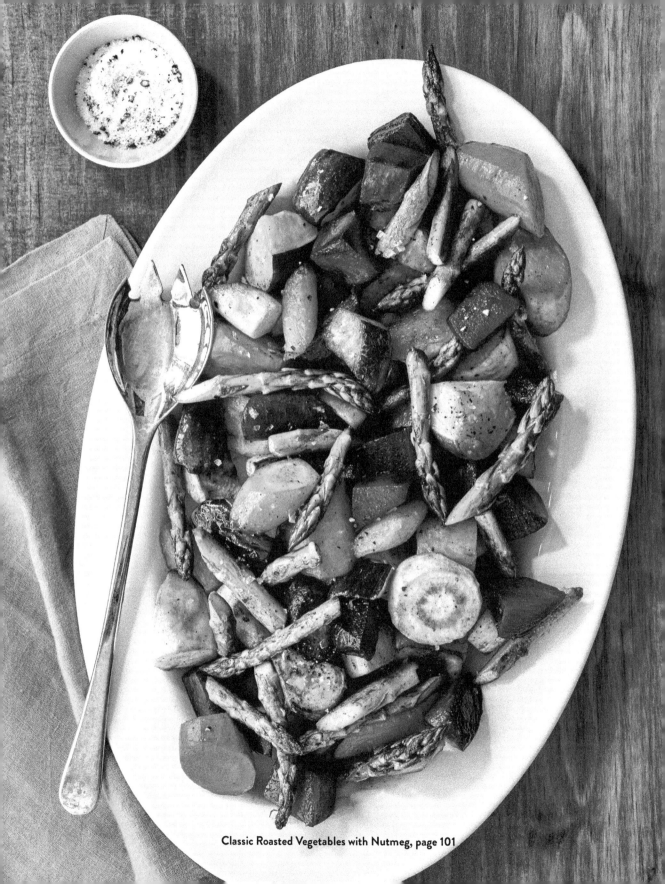

Classic Roasted Vegetables with Nutmeg, page 101

CHAPTER 7

VEGETARIAN & VEGAN MAINS

Black Bean & Sun-Dried Tomato Quesadillas

SERVES 4 / PREP TIME: 20 MINUTES / COOK TIME: 5 MINUTES

30 MINUTES OR LESS, NUT-FREE, UNDER 500 CALORIES, VEGAN

Quesadillas are fun. They are crispy, pretty, and filled with whatever healthy ingredients you have on hand. Black beans are a staple ingredient in Southwestern food and pair well with sweet, sun-dried tomatoes, cool shredded lettuce, and creamy guacamole. Don't let their dark color fool you; black beans are an outstanding source of phytonutrients and are recommended by the American Heart Association as a must-eat food. The soluble fiber in black beans helps you feel full longer while lowering cholesterol levels.

4 (6-inch) whole-wheat tortillas

2 cups canned sodium-free black beans, drained and rinsed

½ cup chopped sun-dried tomatoes

2 scallions, white and green parts, thinly sliced

1 cup shredded romaine lettuce

½ cup Herbed Guacamole (page 167)

1. Preheat the oven to 400°F.

2. Place the tortillas on a baking sheet, and toast them in the oven until crisp, about 5 minutes.

3. While the tortillas are toasting, place the black beans and sun-dried tomatoes in a bowl and mash with a fork.

4. Spread the bean mixture on 2 tortillas and sprinkle with the scallions and lettuce.

5. Spread the guacamole on the remaining 2 tortillas and place them guacamole-side down on the other bean-and-vegetable-topped tortillas. Press together.

6. Cut the quesadillas into quarters and serve two quarters to each person.

Addition Tip: Serve with Classic Roasted Vegetables with Nutmeg (page 101) with a few changes: Omit the nutmeg and add a sprinkle of cumin or coriander to reflect the Southwest theme of the quesadillas. This pairing will increase the calories to 530 per serving.

PER SERVING: Calories: 264; Total fat: 10g; Saturated fat: 1g; Sodium: 321mg; Carbohydrates: 34g; Fiber: 10g; Protein: 13g

Classic Roasted Vegetables with Nutmeg

SERVES 4 / PREP TIME: 20 MINUTES / COOK TIME: 40 MINUTES

ALLERGEN-FREE, DAIRY-FREE, NUT-FREE, UNDER 500 CALORIES, VEGAN

The scent of lightly spiced roasting vegetables with hints of nutmeg and maple, as well as the natural sweetness of root vegetables, will waft throughout your whole house. You might wonder why the beets on the baking tray are segregated on one end. Beets are incredibly healthy but can be very messy to cook; they will stain almost anything they come in contact with, including other vegetables in the recipe and your hands. Wear gloves when you peel them, and if you happen to get stained, rub the areas all over with coarse salt and water and then with mild soap to remove the color.

1 acorn squash, peeled, seeded, and cut into 1-inch cubes

1 celeriac, peeled and cut into 1-inch chunks

2 sweet potatoes, peeled and cut into 1-inch chunks

2 large carrots, cut into 1-inch chunks

2 large parsnips, cut into 1-inch chunks

6 teaspoons olive oil, divided

6 beets, peeled and quartered

1 tablespoon maple syrup

1 teaspoon ground nutmeg

1 bunch asparagus, trimmed and cut into 2-inch pieces

Sea salt

Freshly ground black pepper

1. Preheat the oven to 400°F. Line a baking sheet with foil and set aside.

2. In a large bowl, toss together the squash, celeriac, sweet potatoes, carrots, parsnips, and 4 teaspoons of oil until the vegetables are well coated.

3. Spread the vegetables on two-thirds of the baking sheet.

4. Add the beets to the bowl and toss with 1 teaspoon of oil.

5. Arrange the beets on the baking sheet's remaining space.

6. Drizzle the vegetables with maple syrup and sprinkle with the nutmeg. Place the baking sheet in the oven.

CONTINUED >

7. While the vegetables bake, add the asparagus to the bowl and toss with the remaining 1 teaspoon of oil. Add the asparagus to the baking sheet after the other vegetables have baked for 30 minutes.

8. Continue baking until all the vegetables are lightly caramelized and tender, about 40 minutes total, turning once.

9. Season the vegetables with salt and pepper, toss to combine, and serve.

Addition Tip: Add this gorgeous dish as a side to Honey Sesame Salmon with Bok Choy (page 122) to create a 600-calorie meal. Or add a lightly seasoned chicken breast or pork tenderloin to the baking sheet along with the asparagus to add 150 to 200 calories and create a simple sheet-pan meal.

PER SERVING: Calories: 266; Total fat: 8g; Saturated fat: 1g; Sodium: 127mg; Carbohydrates: 48g; Fiber: 10g; Protein: 6g

Traditional Falafel Pockets

SERVES 4 / PREP TIME: 20 MINUTES / COOK TIME: 25 MINUTES

UNDER 500 CALORIES, VEGAN

Falafel is an ideal meal for fasting because it is filling and nutritious without being packed with calories. Legumes such as chickpeas and nuts are satiating and are rich sources of healthy fats, fiber, and protein. Chickpeas are the traditional base of falafel, but you can use any type of bean—including lentils, navy beans, and cannelloni beans—if you prefer.

1½ cups low-sodium canned chickpeas, drained and rinsed
⅓ sweet onion, chopped
3 tablespoons almond flour
2 teaspoons minced garlic
2 teaspoons chopped fresh parsley
1 teaspoon baking powder
1 teaspoon ground cumin
½ teaspoon ground coriander
Nonstick cooking spray
4 (6-inch) whole-wheat pitas
½ cup Greek yogurt
1 English cucumber, diced
1 large tomato, diced
½ red onion, thinly sliced

1. Preheat the oven to 425°F. Line a baking sheet with parchment paper and set aside.

2. Place the chickpeas, onion, almond flour, garlic, parsley, baking powder, cumin, and coriander in a food processor, and pulse until a soft ball forms.

3. Form the falafel batter into 16 (1½-inch) balls, then flatten them into patties.

4. Lightly spray both sides of each falafel patty with cooking spray, and place on the baking sheet.

5. Bake until the patties are golden and crispy on both sides, about 25 minutes, turning once.

6. Cut the pitas in half and open up the pockets. Stuff the pita halves with 2 patties, and evenly divide the Greek yogurt, cucumber, tomato, and red onion among the 8 halves before serving.

Make Ahead: The chickpea patties can be cooked and individually frozen on a baking sheet, then portioned into freezer bags (two or four per bag). Freeze for up to 2 months, thaw in the refrigerator overnight, and use them as a tasty filling for a quick meal.

PER SERVING: Calories: 275; Total fat: 4g; Saturated fat: 0g; Sodium: 339mg; Carbohydrates: 52g; Fiber: 7g; Protein: 14g

Curried Peanut Vegetable Noodles

SERVES 4 / PREP TIME: 20 MINUTES / COOK TIME: 7 MINUTES

30 MINUTES OR LESS, DAIRY-FREE, ONE POT, UNDER 500 CALORIES, VEGAN

Spiralized vegetables have become so common that you can purchase them in plastic containers in the produce section of the supermarket. You will see carrots, parsnips, and, of course, zucchini in pretty coils waiting for you. Zucchini is a wonderful choice for this recipe because although the peanut sauce is higher in calories, the zucchini is very low in calories, so it evens out. Zucchini is a superb source of potassium and vitamins A and C, can detox the body, and supports a healthy cardiovascular system.

1 tablespoon olive oil

1 cup shredded bok choy

1 cup bean sprouts

1 red bell pepper, thinly sliced

1 yellow bell pepper, thinly sliced

2 scallions, white and green parts, thinly sliced

8 cups spiralized zucchini

½ cup Curried Peanut Sauce (page 164)

1 tablespoon chopped fresh cilantro

½ cup unsalted roasted pumpkin seeds

1. Heat the oil in a large skillet over medium heat.

2. Add the bok choy, bean sprouts, bell peppers, and scallions to the skillet, and sauté until the vegetables are tender, about 5 minutes.

3. Add the zucchini and peanut sauce, and toss until completely warmed through, about 2 minutes.

4. Top with cilantro and pumpkin seeds and serve immediately.

Variation Tip: Use soba noodles or thin udon noodles instead of spiralized zucchini for a more substantial meal. Make the dish ahead of time and let the flavors mellow for at least 4 hours.

PER SERVING: Calories: 281; Total fat: 17g; Saturated fat: 4g; Sodium: 53mg; Carbohydrates: 24g; Fiber: 6g; Protein: 14g

Pumpkin-Kale Tortilla Wraps

**SERVES 4 / PREP TIME: 15 MINUTES, PLUS 15 MINUTES COOLING TIME /
COOK TIME: 25 MINUTES**

NUT-FREE, UNDER 500 CALORIES, VEGAN

Pumpkin is an attractive addition to any recipe but has a real visual impact when you can see its gorgeous color. The pumpkin's bright color indicates its outstanding source of beta-carotene, a potent disease-fighting antioxidant. Pumpkin is also high in fiber, vitamin C, and potassium, making it an essential ingredient for reducing the risk of cancer and inflammation. Sweet potato or yams can be used in these flavorful wraps as well.

1½ cups diced fresh or
   frozen pumpkin
½ tablespoon olive oil
1 red bell pepper, diced
¼ sweet onion, chopped
1 teaspoon minced garlic
1 cup canned low-sodium
   black beans, drained
   and rinsed
½ teaspoon ground cumin
½ teaspoon chili powder
Pinch cayenne pepper
4 (6-inch) whole-grain
   tortillas
2 cups shredded baby kale
4 tablespoons sour cream

1. Place a medium skillet three-quarters full of water on high heat and bring to a boil.

2. Add the pumpkin, reduce the heat to medium, and simmer until the pumpkin is tender, about 10 minutes. Drain and set aside.

3. Heat the oil in a medium skillet over medium-high heat. Sauté the bell pepper, onion, and garlic until softened, about 6 minutes.

4. Add the pumpkin, black beans, cumin, chili powder, and cayenne pepper to the skillet and cook until heated through, about 5 minutes.

5. Remove the mixture from the heat and set aside until cool, about 15 minutes.

6. Spoon the pumpkin filling into the center of each tortilla.

7. Evenly top each tortilla with kale and sour cream.

8. Wrap the tortillas around the filling and serve.

PER SERVING: Calories: 288; Total fat: 9g; Saturated fat: 3g; Sodium: 378mg; Carbohydrates: 45g; Fiber: 12g; Protein: 13g

Parsnip–Sweet Potato Frittata

SERVES 4 / PREP TIME: 15 MINUTES / COOK TIME: 27 MINUTES

UNDER 500 CALORIES, VEGAN

Frittatas are a terrific way to combine ingredients deliciously and attractively to ensure a healthy meal. This frittata includes two types of root vegetables and fiber-packed kale. Parsnips are best purchased after the first frost of fall, and you should look for firm, medium roots with fresh-looking, unblemished skin. Parsnips are low in calories and high in vitamin C, fiber, folate, and manganese.

8 large eggs

¼ cup skim milk or unsweetened almond milk

2 tablespoons chopped fresh basil

Sea salt

Freshly ground black pepper

1 tablespoon olive oil

½ sweet onion, chopped

2 teaspoons minced garlic

2 cups shredded parsnips

2 cups shredded sweet potatoes

1 cup shredded baby kale

1. Preheat the oven to broil.

2. In a medium bowl, whisk together the eggs, milk, and basil. Season with salt and pepper and set aside.

3. Heat the oil in a large oven-safe skillet over medium-high heat.

4. Sauté the onion and garlic until softened, about 3 minutes.

5. Add the parsnips and sweet potatoes and sauté until the vegetables are tender, about 10 minutes.

6. Stir in the kale and sauté for 2 minutes.

7. Pour the egg mixture into the skillet, shaking the pan gently to distribute the egg evenly.

8. As the egg cooks, lift the cooked portions up with a spatula, and let the uncooked egg flow underneath. Cook until the bottom of the frittata is just cooked, about 10 minutes.

9. Broil the frittata until the top is lightly golden and puffy, about 2 minutes.

10. Cut the finished frittata into 4 wedges and serve.

PER SERVING: Calories: 318; Total fat: 12g; Saturated fat: 3g; Sodium: 182mg; Carbohydrates: 37g; Fiber: 8g; Protein: 16g

Wild Rice–Spinach Stew

SERVES 4 / PREP TIME: 15 MINUTES / COOK TIME: 56 MINUTES

ALLERGEN-FREE, DAIRY-FREE, NUT-FREE, ONE POT, UNDER 500 CALORIES, VEGAN

Wild rice is an inspired addition to this vegetable and dark leafy green stew, and its nutty flavor and firm, chewy texture pair well with sweet butternut squash and kidney beans. Wild rice is an aquatic seed that is indigenous to Canada and some northern states, although most products in the grocery store are cultivated rather than picked in the wild. This ingredient is a more nutritious choice than brown or white rice because it is higher in protein, complex carbohydrates, minerals, and vitamin B.

1 tablespoon olive oil

1 sweet onion, chopped

2 celery stalks, chopped

1 tablespoon minced garlic

1 (28-ounce) can low-sodium diced tomatoes

4 cups low-sodium vegetable broth

1 cup wild rice

2 bay leaves

1 cup diced butternut squash

1 cup low-sodium canned red kidney beans, drained and rinsed

4 cups fresh baby spinach

Sea salt

Freshly ground black pepper

2 tablespoons chopped fresh parsley, for garnish

1. Heat the oil in a large stockpot over medium-high heat.

2. Sauté the onion, celery, and garlic until it is softened, about 4 minutes.

3. Stir in the tomatoes, broth, wild rice, and bay leaves and bring to a boil.

4. Reduce the heat to low, and simmer until the rice is almost cooked through, about 40 minutes.

5. Stir in the squash and kidney beans, and simmer for 10 minutes.

6. Remove the bay leaves and stir in the spinach. Simmer for 2 minutes.

7. Season with salt and pepper and serve topped with parsley.

Make Ahead: This is a nice stew to double up and freeze, though omit the spinach until you reheat the dish.

PER SERVING: Calories: 328; Total fat: 4g; Saturated fat: 1g; Sodium: 296mg; Carbohydrates: 56g; Fiber: 10g; Protein: 17g

Grain-&-Tofu-Stuffed Eggplant with Tahini

SERVES 4 / PREP TIME: 20 MINUTES / COOK TIME: 25 MINUTES

DAIRY-FREE, NUT-FREE, UNDER 500 CALORIES, VEGAN

Recipes such as this one requires that you press the tofu to remove liquid, so it stays intact during the cooking process. If you'd like to make the grains ahead of time, cook the bulger (1:2 ratio of grains to water) for 12 minutes and see the tip (page 83) for cooking quinoa.

2 small eggplants

2 tablespoons olive oil, divided

½ sweet onion, chopped

1 tablespoon minced garlic

8 ounces extra-firm tofu, pressed and diced into ½-inch cubes

1 cup cooked bulgur

1 cup cooked quinoa

1 cup quartered cherry tomatoes

2 tablespoons tahini

2 tablespoons chopped fresh parsley

Juice of ½ lemon

1. Cut the eggplants in half and scoop out the flesh until about 1-inch thickness remains. Reserve the flesh for another recipe.

2. Preheat the oven to 425°F.

3. Place the eggplants on a baking sheet, hollow-side up, and drizzle with 1 tablespoon of oil. Bake until tender, about 15 minutes.

4. While the eggplant is cooking, heat the remaining 1 tablespoon of oil in a large skillet over medium-high heat.

5. Sauté the onion and garlic until softened, about 3 minutes.

6. Add the tofu and sauté until browned on all sides, about 5 minutes.

7. Remove the skillet from the heat and stir in the bulgur, quinoa, tomatoes, tahini, parsley, and lemon juice until well mixed.

8. Reduce the oven temperature to 350°F and stuff each eggplant half with the grain and tofu mixture. Bake for another 10 minutes before serving.

PER SERVING: Calories: 334; Total fat: 15g; Saturated fat: 2g; Sodium: 65mg; Carbohydrates: 39g; Fiber: 12g; Protein: 15g

Pecan-Tofu Noodle Salad

**SERVES 4 / PREP TIME: 20 MINUTES / COOK TIME: 9 MINUTES,
PLUS 4 HOURS CHILL TIME**

30 MINUTES OR LESS, DAIRY-FREE, UNDER 500 CALORIES, VEGAN

If you are a fan of Asian-style dishes, these spicy, coconut-infused noodles and vegetables will delight your senses. The crunch of rich, chopped pecans adds another layer of texture to the already complex taste experience. Soba noodles are the base in the recipe, and their strong flavor comes from buckwheat flour. Soba noodles are very high in protein as well as B vitamins and can help lower cholesterol and blood pressure.

6 ounces soba noodles

2 carrots, shredded

1 red bell pepper,
    thinly sliced

1 cup julienned snow peas

2 scallions, white and
    green parts, cut into
    julienne strips
    approximately
    2 inches long

½ cup chopped pecans

¼ cup sesame oil

¼ cup light coconut milk

2 tablespoons
    tamari sauce

2 teaspoons ground
    coriander

1 teaspoon hot chili oil

1 tablespoon chopped
    fresh cilantro,
    for garnish

1. Place a medium saucepan filled about three-quarters with water over high heat and bring to a boil.

2. Cook the soba noodles until al dente, about 5 minutes, drain, and rinse under cold water.

3. Transfer the noodles to a large bowl and add the carrots, bell pepper, snow peas, scallions, and pecans. Toss to combine and set aside.

4. In a small bowl, stir together the sesame oil, coconut milk, tamari sauce, coriander, and chili oil.

5. Add the dressing to the salad, stir to coat, and chill the mixture in the refrigerator, covered, for 4 hours.

6. Serve topped with cilantro.

Make Ahead: Cook the soba noodles, drain, rinse, cool, and store in a zip-top bag with the air squeezed out. They will keep in the refrigerator for up to 3 days.

PER SERVING: Calories: 355; Total fat: 18g; Saturated fat: 3g; Sodium: 632mg; Carbohydrates: 42g; Fiber: 5g; Protein: 11g

Tofu Moussaka

SERVES 4 / PREP TIME: 15 MINUTES / COOK TIME: 50 MINUTES

NUT-FREE, UNDER 500 CALORIES, VEGAN

Moussaka is a Middle Eastern dish that features eggplant and rich calorie-laden béchamel sauce. This version is topped by lighter yogurt and ricotta cheese, so it can be a delicious part of a fasting diet. Eggplant is a marvelous source of fiber, copper, manganese, and vitamin B6, as well as antioxidants including zeaxanthin, nasunin, and lutein. The fiber in eggplant can help manage weight because it helps you feel full longer; you won't be tempted to snack or overeat later.

2 tablespoons olive oil, divided, plus extra for greasing

1 sweet onion, chopped

2 teaspoons minced garlic

1 pound diced extra-firm tofu

1 (28-ounce) can low-sodium crushed tomatoes

2 tablespoons chopped fresh basil

2 large eggplants, cut into ½-inch-thick disks

1 cup plain Greek yogurt

1 cup ricotta cheese

Sea salt

Freshly ground black pepper

1. Preheat the oven to 425°F. Lightly grease a 9-by-13-inch baking dish with oil and set aside.

2. Heat 1 tablespoon of oil in a large saucepan over medium-high heat.

3. Sauté the onion and garlic until softened, about 3 minutes. Stir in the tofu, tomatoes, and basil, and bring the sauce to a boil, then reduce the heat to low and simmer until the sauce is thickened, about 20 minutes.

4. While the sauce is simmering, heat the remaining 1 tablespoon of oil in a large skillet over medium-high heat and fry the eggplant slices in batches until browned, about 10 minutes, turning once. Place the fried slices on a paper towel to blot the oil.

5. When the sauce is finished, layer it with the eggplant slices in the baking dish starting with the sauce and ending with the eggplant, about four layers in total.

6. In a small bowl, whisk together the yogurt and ricotta and season with salt and pepper.

7. Spread the yogurt mixture over the eggplant, and bake the casserole until lightly browned, about 25 minutes. Serve.

Substitution Tip: If you do not need a vegetarian meal, use ¾ pound of extra-lean ground beef in place of the tofu. This change will add 70 calories and 10 grams of protein per serving.

PER SERVING: Calories: 389; Total fat: 18g; Saturated fat: 7g; Sodium: 287mg; Carbohydrates: 39g; Fiber: 11g; Protein: 22g

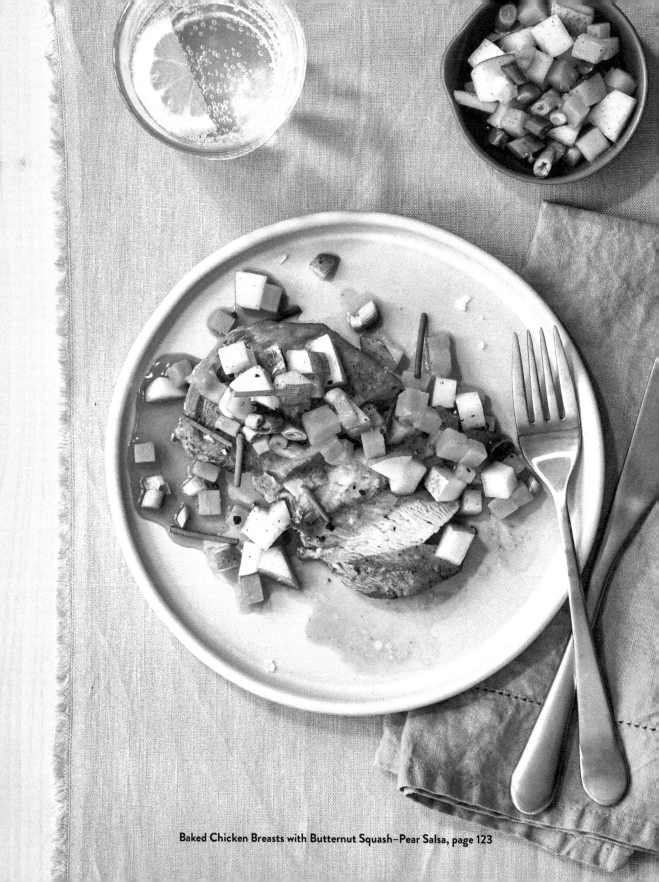

Baked Chicken Breasts with Butternut Squash–Pear Salsa, page 123

CHAPTER 8

POULTRY & SEAFOOD MAINS

Skillet Asian Chicken Breasts

SERVES 4 / PREP TIME: 15 MINUTES / COOK TIME: 20 MINUTES

DAIRY-FREE, UNDER 500 CALORIES

Chicken breast is a very popular choice in healthy diets because it is an excellent source of protein and a very good source of B vitamins, niacin, phosphorus, and selenium. Chicken can help boost metabolism, build or maintain muscle, and support healthy blood vessels. Make sure your chicken breasts are not pumped with saline (read the label), so you don't get an unwanted influx of sodium.

½ cup low-sodium chicken broth

1 tablespoon coconut aminos or tamari sauce

1 tablespoon honey

1 tablespoon cornstarch

2 teaspoons peeled, grated fresh ginger

1 teaspoon minced garlic

1 tablespoon olive oil

16 ounces boneless, skinless chicken breast, cut into 1-inch cubes

2 cups shredded bok choy

1 red bell pepper, thinly sliced

1 tablespoon sesame seeds, for garnish

1. In a small bowl, stir together the broth, coconut aminos, honey, cornstarch, ginger, and garlic and set sauce aside.

2. Heat the oil in a large skillet over medium-high heat.

3. Sauté the chicken breast until it is just cooked through and lightly browned, 12 to 15 minutes.

4. Add the bok choy and bell pepper, and sauté for 5 minutes more.

5. Push the chicken and vegetables to the side of the skillet and pour in the sauce.

6. Cook, stirring frequently, until the sauce has thickened, 3 to 4 minutes.

7. Toss the chicken and vegetables with the sauce.

8. Serve topped with sesame seeds.

Addition Tip: Serve with Pecan-Tofu Noodle Salad (page 109) for a meal that has 563 calories, or the Kale Salad with Peach & Blue Cheese (page 92) for a 499-calorie pairing. The chicken breast can be used cold in wraps, salads, and casseroles when you want a little extra flavor and protein.

PER SERVING: Calories: 208; Total fat: 6g; Saturated fat: 1g; Sodium: 112mg; Carbohydrates: 11g; Fiber: 1g; Protein: 28g

Cajun-Style Fish-Tomato Stew

SERVES 4 / PREP TIME: 20 MINUTES / COOK TIME: 35 MINUTES

DAIRY-FREE, NUT-FREE, ONE POT, UNDER 500 CALORIES

Fish stews are found in many countries around the world and are obviously most popular in areas that border large bodies of water such as oceans, lakes, and rivers. This recipe takes its inspiration from the South, with Louisiana-style spices and a lot of hearty vegetables. The fish is added at the end of the cooking process, so look for a mild "unfishy" choice such as tilapia, cod, or halibut for the best flavor.

1 tablespoon olive oil

1 sweet onion, chopped

1 green bell pepper, diced

3 celery stalks, sliced

1 tablespoon minced garlic

1 tablespoon Cajun seasoning

1 (15-ounce) can low-sodium diced tomatoes

1 cup low-sodium chicken broth

4 (5-ounce) boneless, skinless firm fish, cut into 1-inch pieces

1 cup shredded carrot

1 cup shredded Swiss chard

1 tablespoon chopped fresh parsley, for garnish

1. Heat the oil in a large saucepan over medium-high heat.

2. Sauté the onion, bell pepper, celery, and garlic until softened, about 5 minutes.

3. Stir in the seasoning and sauté for 2 minutes more.

4. Stir in the tomatoes and broth and bring the mixture to a boil.

5. Reduce the heat to medium-low and simmer for 15 minutes.

6. Stir in the fish and carrot and simmer until the fish is just cooked through, 7 to 8 minutes.

7. Remove from the heat, stir in the Swiss chard, and let the stew sit for 5 minutes to wilt the greens.

8. Serve topped with parsley.

Addition Tip: This spicy creation is thick enough to be served over a cooked grain such as quinoa or brown rice. One cup of cooked brown rice will bump the calories to 427 per serving.

PER SERVING: Calories: 211; Total fat: 5g; Saturated fat: 1g; Sodium: 219mg; Carbohydrates: 14g; Fiber: 3g; Protein: 28g

Hearty Turkey-Vegetable Stew

SERVES 4 / PREP TIME: 20 MINUTES/ COOK TIME: 35 MINUTES

Turkey sits right next to the chicken in the produce section of your supermarket, but unless a major holiday is on the calendar, you probably pass it by. Next time you are shopping, pick up a turkey breast and use it for some of your favorite recipes, like this pleasing stew. Turkey is a terrific source of protein, iron, potassium, and niacin. It is also low in calories if skinless, so it is ideal for weight loss.

1 tablespoon olive oil

16 ounces boneless, skinless turkey breast, cut into ½-inch chunks

1 sweet onion, chopped

3 celery stalks, chopped

2 teaspoons minced garlic

6 cups low-sodium chicken broth

1 cup shredded cabbage

1 cup small cauliflower florets

2 carrots, thinly sliced

1 zucchini, diced

1 yellow bell pepper, diced

Pinch red pepper flakes

Sea salt

Freshly ground black pepper

2 tablespoons chopped fresh parsley, for garnish

1. Heat the oil in a large stockpot over medium-high heat.

2. Sauté the turkey until browned and cooked halfway through, about 10 minutes.

3. Add the onion, celery, and garlic and cook until softened, about 5 minutes.

4. Stir in the broth, cabbage, cauliflower, and carrots, and bring the mixture to a boil.

5. Reduce the heat to low, and simmer until the vegetables are tender and the turkey is cooked through, about 15 minutes.

6. Stir in the zucchini, bell pepper, and red pepper flakes, and simmer for 5 minutes more.

7. Season the stew with salt and pepper.

8. Serve topped with parsley.

Substitution Tip: Omit the turkey and use vegetable broth for a vegan version of this filling stew. Add canned legumes such as lentils, white beans, or split peas instead of the poultry for bulk.

PER SERVING: Calories: 230; Total fat: 4g; Saturated fat: 1g; Sodium: 155mg; Carbohydrates: 15g; Fiber: 4g; Protein: 33g

Chicken & Sweet Potato with Peaches

SERVES 4 / PREP TIME: 15 MINUTES / COOK TIME: 37 MINUTES

ALLERGEN-FREE, DAIRY-FREE, NUT-FREE, ONE POT, UNDER 500 CALORIES

Chicken enhanced by sweet stone fruit, such as apricots or peaches, is a popular North African dish, especially when mixed with warm spices like ginger and cinnamon. Peel the peaches to create a smooth texture; to do this, place the fruit in boiling water until the skin splits, about 15 to 20 seconds, then dunk them in cold water and use a paring knife to slip the skins off.

1 tablespoon olive oil

16 ounces boneless, skinless chicken breast, cut into 1-inch chunks

½ sweet onion, chopped

2 teaspoons minced garlic

2 teaspoons peeled grated fresh ginger

1 teaspoon ground cinnamon

½ teaspoon ground nutmeg

1 cup low-sodium chicken broth, divided

Juice of 1 orange

1 sweet potato, peeled and diced

1 tablespoon cornstarch

2 peaches, peeled, pitted, and diced

1 teaspoon chopped fresh thyme

1. Heat the oil in a large skillet over medium-high heat.

2. Sauté the chicken until just cooked through and lightly browned, about 10 minutes. Set aside.

3. Add the onion, garlic, ginger, cinnamon, and nutmeg, and sauté until the vegetables are softened, about 3 minutes.

4. Return the chicken to the skillet along with ¾ cup of broth, orange juice, and sweet potato.

5. Bring the mixture to a boil, then reduce heat to medium-low and simmer the stew until the sweet potato and chicken are tender, about 20 minutes.

6. Stir the cornstarch into the remaining ¼ cup of broth and add the mixture and peaches to the skillet.

7. Simmer until the stew thickens, about 4 minutes.

8. Stir in the thyme and serve.

Craving Tip: Peaches and orange juice add sweetness satisfying any sugar cravings. Add a mixed green salad or tender cooked grains such as wheat berries or quinoa to round out the meal.

PER SERVING: Calories: 240; Total fat: 5g; Saturated fat: 1g; Sodium: 112mg; Carbohydrates: 21g; Fiber: 3g; Protein: 28g

Pan-Seared Trout with Dill & Leeks

SERVES 4 / PREP TIME: 15 MINUTES / COOK TIME: 20 MINUTES

DAIRY-FREE, NUT-FREE, ONE POT, UNDER 500 CALORIES

Leeks are an elegant vegetable, slender and ombré in color from creamy white to deep green. They have a milder flavor than regular onions and look bright and fresh when sautéed with fragrant garlic. Leeks need to be thoroughly cleaned after they are sliced because dirt can cake among their many layers. Soak the leek slices in a bowl of cold water, swirling them around and then letting them sit for 10 to 15 minutes. The dirt will settle to the bottom of the bowl, and you can scoop the clean, floating vegetable slices from the surface.

1 tablespoon olive oil

3 leeks, green and white parts, thinly sliced

1 tablespoon minced garlic

4 (5-ounce) boneless, skinless trout fillets

Sea salt

Freshly ground black pepper

¼ cup low-sodium chicken broth

2 teaspoons chopped fresh dill, for garnish

1. Heat the oil in a large skillet over medium-high heat.

2. Sauté the leeks and garlic until tender, about 10 minutes.

3. Lightly season the fish with salt and pepper and place the fillets in the skillet with the vegetables.

4. Add the broth, cover, and reduce the heat to medium-low.

5. Cook until the fish flakes easily with a fork, about 10 minutes, depending on the thickness.

6. Serve topped with dill.

Addition Tip: This simple dish can be paired with almost any other recipe to create a full-calorie meal. Try Fresh Green Bean Salad with Herbs (page 156) or mixed vegetables sautéed in a little butter for a summer-inspired meal.

PER SERVING: Calories: 254, Total fat: 11g; Saturated fat: 1g; Sodium: 78mg; Carbohydrates: 11g; Fiber: 1g; Protein: 29g

Baked Haddock-Mushroom Casserole

SERVES 4 / PREP TIME: 15 MINUTES / COOK TIME: 36 MINUTES

DAIRY-FREE, NUT-FREE, ONE POT, UNDER 500 CALORIES

Cauliflower takes the place of grain in this nourishing casserole, which adds many important nutrients to the meal. This vegetable is rich in fiber; vitamins A, C, and K; omega-3 essential fatty acids; manganese; and potassium. Cauliflower can lower your risk of cancer, inflammatory diseases, and cardiovascular disease. You can either chop the cauliflower yourself or purchase riced cauliflower in the produce section of the grocery store to save a bit of preparation time.

1 tablespoon olive oil

2 cups sliced mushrooms

1 sweet onion, chopped

2 teaspoons minced garlic

2 cups finely chopped cauliflower

1 cup low-sodium chicken broth

2 tablespoons tomato paste

1 pound haddock, cut into 1-inch chunks

1 (15-ounce) can low-sodium lentils, drained and rinsed

Sea salt

Freshly ground black pepper

1 tablespoon chopped fresh thyme, for garnish

1. Preheat the oven to 350°F.

2. Heat the oil in a large oven-safe skillet over medium-high heat.

3. Sauté the mushrooms, onion, and garlic until the mushrooms are lightly caramelized, about 10 minutes.

4. Stir in the cauliflower, and sauté for 2 minutes more.

5. Stir in the broth and tomato paste until well combined, and bring the liquid to a boil, about 4 minutes.

6. Add the fish and lentils, cover, and bake in the oven until the fish is just cooked through, about 20 minutes.

7. Season with salt and pepper and serve topped with thyme.

Substitution Tip: The fish can be replaced with extra-firm tofu and the broth swapped for vegetable broth to create a vegan meal. Make sure you press the tofu and sauté it with the mushrooms until lightly browned before adding to the casserole.

PER SERVING: Calories: 272; Total fat: 5g; Saturated fat: 1g; Sodium: 354mg; Carbohydrates: 29g; Fiber: 11g; Protein: 30g

Market Bulgur-Chicken Skillet

SERVES 4 / PREP TIME: 20 MINUTES / COOK TIME: 20 MINUTES

ALLERGEN-FREE, DAIRY-FREE, NUT-FREE, UNDER 500 CALORIES

Simple is sometimes very effective when you are working with whole foods such as lean chicken breast, fresh produce, and healthy grains like bulgur. Bulgur is dried, cracked durum wheat that is partially cooked (parboiled) so that it can be prepared quickly. This whole grain is high in vitamin E, fiber, protein, potassium, magnesium, and folate, so it can reduce the risk of diabetes and cardiovascular disease.

1 cup low-sodium chicken broth
½ cup bulgur
1 tablespoon olive oil
12 ounces boneless, skinless chicken breast, cut into ½-inch wide slices
1 sweet onion, chopped
1 tablespoon minced garlic
1 zucchini, halved lengthwise and cut into half disks
1 red bell pepper, thinly sliced
1 cup fresh or frozen corn kernels
1 cup green beans, cut into 1-inch pieces
1 cup low-sodium canned lentils, drained and rinsed
1 tablespoon chopped fresh basil
Juice and zest of 1 lemon
Sea salt
Freshly ground black pepper

1. Place a medium saucepan over medium-high heat and add the broth and bulgur.

2. Bring the mixture to a boil, then reduce the heat to low and simmer until the grain is tender, about 12 minutes.

3. While the bulgur is cooking, heat the oil in a large skillet over medium-high heat.

4. Sauté the chicken until it is just cooked through and lightly browned, about 10 minutes.

5. Remove the chicken with a slotted spoon to a plate and set aside.

6. Add the onion and garlic to the skillet, and sauté until softened, about 3 minutes.

7. Add the zucchini, bell pepper, corn, green beans, and lentils to the skillet, and sauté until the vegetables are tender-crisp, about 7 minutes.

8. Stir in the bulgur, chicken, basil, and lemon juice and zest.

9. Season with salt and pepper and serve.

- -

Make Ahead: Cook the bulgur a couple of days in advance (see tip page 108), and use cooked chicken for a quick, convenient meal. Try a simple rotisserie chicken with the skin removed for added flavor.

PER SERVING: Calories: 315; Total fat: 6g; Saturated fat: 1g; Sodium: 93mg; Carbohydrates: 40g; Fiber: 11g; Protein: 30g

Honey Sesame Salmon with Bok Choy

SERVES 4 / PREP TIME: 10 MINUTES / COOK TIME: 20 MINUTES

30 MINUTES OR LESS, DAIRY-FREE, NUT-FREE, ONE POT, UNDER 500 CALORIES

You can have this wholesome, attractive dish on the table in about half an hour, and since the fish cooks with its own side dish, you have even less work to do! The most arduous part of the preparation is cleaning the bok choy so the dirt at the base doesn't end up in the dish. The sweet honey and toasty sesame seeds offset the slight bitterness of the bok choy, creating culinary perfection.

4 (4-ounce) salmon fillets
Sea salt
Freshly ground
  black pepper
1 teaspoon sesame oil
2 tablespoons honey
2 tablespoons
  sesame seeds
¼ cup low-sodium
  chicken broth
4 cups shredded bok choy

1. Preheat the oven to 450°F.

2. Lightly season the salmon with salt and pepper.

3. Heat the oil in a large oven-safe skillet over medium-high heat.

4. Pan-sear the salmon on both sides until lightly browned, about 10 minutes, turning once.

5. Spread the honey on top of the salmon, and sprinkle with the sesame seeds. Move the fillets to one side of the skillet.

6. Pour the broth in the skillet and add the bok choy to the other side of the skillet.

7. Cover and place the skillet in the oven until the fish is just cooked through and the bok choy is tender, 8 to 10 minutes.

8. Season the bok choy with salt and pepper and serve.

Addition Tip: Serve this dish with Grain-&-Tofu-Stuffed Eggplant with Tahini (page 108) as a side dish to create a 650-calorie combination. The tahini-flavored sauce can be drizzled over the bok choy as well.

PER SERVING: Calories: 317; Total fat: 16g; Saturated fat: 4g; Sodium: 127mg; Carbohydrates: 11g; Fiber: 1g; Protein: 26g

Baked Chicken Breasts with Butternut Squash–Pear Salsa

**SERVES 4 / PREP TIME: 15 MINUTES, PLUS 15 MINUTES COOLING TIME /
COOK TIME: 35 MINUTES**

ALLERGEN-FREE, DAIRY-FREE, NUT-FREE, UNDER 500 CALORIES

Sometimes the topping or sauce in a dish is the star and the proteins are just the base to highlight it. This salsa is incredibly bright, sweet, and complex with spices and rich maple syrup. Butternut squash is a fruit and a member of the gourd family. It is low-fat, fiber-packed, and high in heart-healthy carotenoids. When you add firm pears, the filling fiber content is even higher. Keep the skin on the pears because this part of the fruit contains the majority of disease-fighting phytonutrients. Wash the pears thoroughly with a soft brush to remove any pesticides or contaminants from the skin.

½ butternut squash, peeled, seeded, and diced into ¼-inch cubes

2 tablespoons olive oil, divided

½ teaspoon ground nutmeg

¼ teaspoon ground cinnamon

2 pears, cored and diced

1 scallion, white and green parts, finely chopped

1 tablespoon maple syrup

Juice of 1 lime

Sea salt

Freshly ground black pepper

4 (4-ounce) boneless, skinless chicken breasts

1. Preheat the oven to 400°F. Line a baking sheet with foil and set aside.

2. In a small bowl, toss the squash with 1 tablespoon of oil, the nutmeg, and cinnamon.

3. Spread the squash on the baking sheet and roast, stirring once, until lightly caramelized but not mushy, about 15 minutes.

4. Transfer the roasted squash to a medium bowl, and let it cool for 15 minutes.

5. Stir in the pears, scallion, maple syrup, and lime juice. Season with salt and pepper, and set aside.

CONTINUED >

6. Heat the remaining 1 tablespoon of oil in a large skillet over medium-high heat and lightly season the chicken with salt and pepper.

7. Panfry the chicken breasts until completely cooked through, turning once, until the internal temperature is 165°F, about 20 minutes.

8. Serve the chicken with salsa.

Make Ahead: The salsa can be made 2 to 3 days ahead and stored in the refrigerator. Just leave it out until it is room temperature, or gently warm the salsa in a small skillet before topping the chicken.

PER SERVING: Calories: 322; Total fat: 9g; Saturated fat: 1g; Sodium: 83mg; Carbohydrates: 37g; Fiber: 7g; Protein: 28g

Mediterranean Fish Tacos

SERVES 4 / PREP TIME: 25 MINUTES / COOK TIME: 10 MINUTES

NUT-FREE, UNDER 500 CALORIES

Fish tacos usually feature Southwest-style ingredients, but the fresh vegetables, olives, and feta cheese associated with the Mediterranean region work well, too. Black olives, such as Kalamata, are high in healthy monounsaturated fat, iron, and vitamin E, so they can help prevent blood clots and lower cholesterol. Olives are brined and can be high in sodium, so enjoy them in moderate quantities.

1 pound firm white fish (cod, tilapia, or catfish), cut into 4 pieces

Sea salt

Freshly ground black pepper

1 teaspoon dried oregano

½ teaspoon dried basil

1 tablespoon olive oil

4 corn taco shells

1 English cucumber, chopped

1 cup chopped tomatoes

½ cup Kalamata olives, sliced

½ cup crumbled low-sodium feta cheese

2 cups shredded baby kale

1. Lightly season the fish with salt and pepper. Sprinkle with the oregano and basil.

2. Heat the oil in a large skillet over medium-high heat. Cook the fish until just cooked through, turning once, about 10 minutes.

3. Place one piece of fish in each taco shell, and evenly divide the cucumber, tomatoes, olives, cheese, and kale among the shells before serving.

Addition Tip: Add a few generous spoonfuls of Herbed Guacamole (page 167) as a tasty topping on these colorful tacos. This addition will bump the calories per serving to 458.

PER SERVING: Calories: 359; Total fat: 14g; Saturated fat: 7g; Sodium: 509mg; Carbohydrates: 24g; Fiber: 5g; Protein: 27g

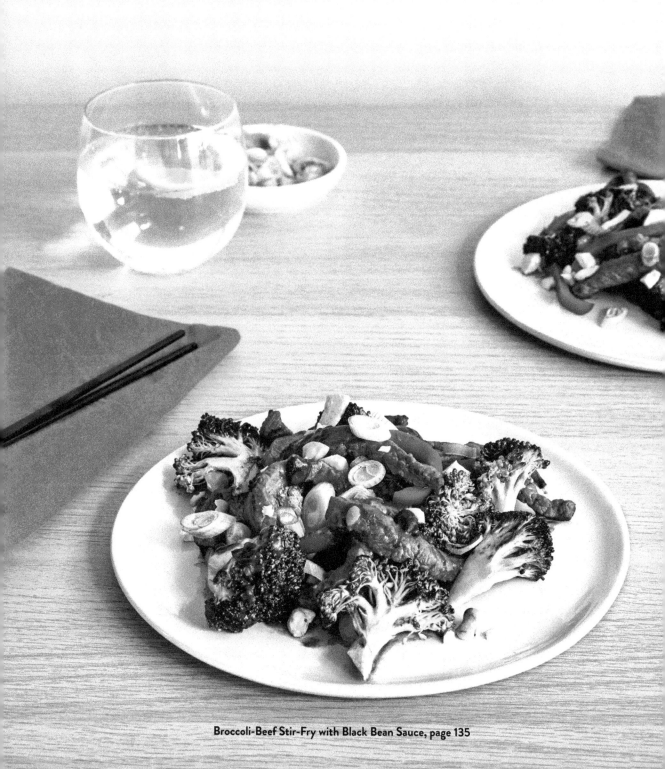

Broccoli-Beef Stir-Fry with Black Bean Sauce, page 135

CHAPTER 9

BEEF & PORK MAINS

Pork Tenderloin Medallions with Herb Sauce

SERVES 4 / PREP TIME: 15 MINUTES / COOK TIME: 17 MINUTES

DAIRY-FREE, UNDER 500 CALORIES

Pork tenderloin is a melt-in-your-mouth tender cut of meat that is low in calories but high in protein. Farmers in the United States are actually given incentives to produce lean animals, so you can be assured your meal is weight-loss friendly. These almond-breaded cutlets soak up the herb-infused sauce and create a flavorful dish. Try any type of ground nut as the breading, or panko bread crumbs if you want to boost the calories.

½ cup almond flour
Pinch sea salt
Pinch freshly ground
  black pepper
1 pound pork tenderloin,
  cut into 3-inch-thick
  pieces, pounded to
  ½-inch-thick medallions
2 tablespoons olive oil
½ cup low-sodium
  chicken stock
Juice and zest of 1 lemon
1 teaspoon chopped
  fresh parsley
1 teaspoon chopped
  fresh thyme

1. In a small bowl, combine the almond flour, salt, and pepper.

2. Dredge the pork medallions in the almond flour mixture and set aside.

3. Heat the oil in a large skillet over medium-high heat.

4. Add the pork and panfry until browned and cooked through, about 12 minutes, turning once.

5. Remove the pork to a plate, cover with foil, and set aside.

6. Add the chicken stock to the skillet, stirring to scrape up any meaty bits, and simmer until the liquid is reduced by half, about 5 minutes.

7. Stir in the lemon juice, zest, parsley, and thyme.

8. Add the pork back to the skillet, turning to coat the pork in the sauce, and serve warm.

Addition Tip: Serve with Classic Roasted Vegetables with Nutmeg (page 101), or grill oil-tossed bell peppers, zucchini, and asparagus. The vegetable combination will add 150 to 200 calories per serving.

PER SERVING: Calories: 226; Total fat: 14g;
Saturated fat: 2g; Sodium: 312mg; Carbohydrates: 2g;
Fiber: 1g; Protein: 23g

Broiled Beef Tenderloin with Maple Barbecue Sauce

SERVES 4 / PREP TIME: 10 MINUTES / COOK TIME: 10 MINUTES, PLUS 10 MINUTES RESTING TIME

5 INGREDIENTS OR LESS, 30 MINUTES OR LESS, ALLERGEN-FREE, DAIRY-FREE, NUT-FREE, ONE POT, UNDER 500 CALORIES

Beef can be a good choice on a weight-loss diet if you prepare a lean cut, about 4 grams of fat per 3-ounce portion, such as beef tenderloin. Make sure you trim off any visible fat to ensure this ratio. Beef is packed with satiating protein and nutrients such as iron, vitamin B12, and zinc. Trimmed sirloin steak is also delicious in this dish.

4 (4-ounce) beef tenderloin medallions
Sea salt
Freshly ground black pepper
1 tablespoon olive oil
½ cup Maple Barbecue Sauce (page 162), divided

1. Preheat the oven to broil.

2. Lightly season the beef all over with salt and pepper.

3. Heat the oil in a large oven-safe skillet over high heat.

4. Pan-sear the beef on all sides until completely browned, 6 to 8 minutes. Baste the beef with ¼ cup of barbecue sauce, and broil until desired doneness, about 10 minutes for medium-rare (120°F to 125°F on a meat thermometer), turning once.

5. Let the meat rest for 10 minutes and baste with the remaining ¼ cup of sauce before serving.

Addition Tip: Try Fresh Green Bean Salad with Herbs (page 156) to complement this perfect, simple meal. This combination will give you 471 calories per serving and a satisfying balance of protein and complex carbohydrates.

PER SERVING: Calories: 229; Total fat: 10g; Saturated fat: 3g; Sodium: 143mg; Carbohydrates: 6g; Fiber: 1g; Protein: 26g

Fiery Pork Lettuce Wraps

SERVES 4 / PREP TIME: 20 MINUTES / COOK TIME: 20 MINUTES

ALLERGEN-FREE, DAIRY-FREE, NUT-FREE, UNDER 500 CALORIES

Lettuce might seem like just the container for the tasty spiced filling in this dish, but it adds nutrition and fresh complementary flavor as well. Lettuce is rich in potassium and vitamins A and K. Some good options for wraps could be Boston lettuce, which has large tender leaves or romaine, which is firmer but the thick rib down the middle of the leaf needs to be removed for easier rolling.

For the sauce:

¼ cup low-sodium chicken broth
1 tablespoon rice vinegar
1 tablespoon honey
1 teaspoon hoisin sauce
1 teaspoon cornstarch
1 teaspoon tamari sauce
Pinch red pepper flakes

For the wraps:

1 teaspoon sesame oil
1 pound lean ground pork
1 teaspoon minced garlic
2 carrots, shredded
1 red bell pepper, thinly sliced
1 yellow bell pepper, thinly sliced
1 cup shredded Napa cabbage
1 scallion, white and green parts, thinly sliced
8 large lettuce leaves

To make the sauce:

In a small bowl, whisk together the broth, vinegar, honey, hoisin sauce, cornstarch, tamari sauce, and red pepper flakes. Set aside.

To make the wraps:

1. Heat the oil in a large skillet over medium-high heat.

2. Sauté the pork and garlic until the meat is cooked through, about 8 minutes.

3. Add the carrots, bell peppers, cabbage, and scallion to the skillet, and sauté until the vegetables are tender, about 7 minutes.

4. Move the pork and vegetable mixture to one side of the skillet and pour in the sauce.

5. Stir the sauce until it thickens, about 5 minutes.

6. Combine the meat and vegetables with the sauce and remove the skillet from the heat.

7. Spoon the hot pork filling into the lettuce leaves and serve.

Make Ahead: The filling can be made 1 to 2 days prior and stored in the refrigerator. Double up on the pork mixture to use as a protein-rich topping on salads or over cooked brown rice.

PER SERVING: Calories: 259; Total fat: 11g; Saturated fat: 4g; Sodium: 206mg; Carbohydrates: 16g; Fiber: 2g; Protein: 24g

Rich Pork Stroganoff

SERVES 4 / PREP TIME: 15 MINUTES / COOK TIME: 38 MINUTES

NUT-FREE, UNDER 500 CALORIES

Tender chunks of pork showcase luscious mushroom-studded sauce with the pleasing richness of sour cream. The combination is delectable even though this recipe is usually prepared with beef strips. Sour cream is created by mixing heavy cream with bacteria, so the mixture thickens and becomes tangy. Look for sour cream that contains probiotics so you enjoy the benefit of improved digestion.

1 tablespoon olive oil

1 pound pork tenderloin, cut into ½-inch cubes

2 cups sliced mushrooms

1 sweet onion, thinly sliced

1 tablespoon minced garlic

1 cup low-sodium chicken broth

1 (15-ounce) can low-sodium crushed tomatoes

1 tablespoon smoked paprika

½ cup sour cream or plain Greek yogurt

Sea salt

Freshly ground black pepper

2 tablespoons chopped fresh parsley, for garnish

1. Heat the oil in a large skillet over medium-high heat.

2. Sauté the pork until just cooked through and lightly browned, about 10 minutes. Remove the cooked pork to a plate with a slotted spoon, cover with foil, and set aside.

3. Add the mushrooms, onion, and garlic to the skillet, and sauté until the mushrooms are lightly caramelized, about 8 minutes.

4. Stir in the reserved pork, broth, tomatoes, and paprika, and bring the sauce to a boil.

5. Reduce the heat to low, and simmer until the meat is very tender and the sauce reduces by about one-quarter, 18 to 20 minutes.

6. Remove from the heat and stir in the sour cream.

7. Season with salt and pepper and serve topped with parsley.

Addition Tip: Serve over cooked grains such as brown rice, bulgur, or whole-grain noodles if you want a more traditional meal. The delicious sauce soaks in beautifully, and you won't waste a single spoonful.

PER SERVING: Calories: 263; Total fat: 13g; Saturated fat: 5g; Sodium: 145mg; Carbohydrates: 11g; Fiber: 2g; Protein: 24g

Beef-&-Farro-Stuffed Peppers

SERVES 4 / PREP TIME: 15 MINUTES / COOK TIME: 1 HOUR

NUT-FREE, UNDER 500 CALORIES

Stuffed veggies are a charming addition to any meal because they look attractive and the filling is neatly contained in the peppers, tomatoes, zucchini, or squash. This recipe uses sweet bell peppers, and the filling is a classic beef, grain, and spinach mixture. Avoid buying spinach stored in a dark section of the store. Spinach has more nutrients when in direct sunlight, even in a plastic bag.

1 tablespoon olive oil, plus more for greasing

4 large bell peppers, any color

½ pound extra-lean ground beef

1 sweet onion, chopped

1 cup shredded carrot

2 teaspoons minced garlic

1 cup chopped fresh baby spinach

1 cup cooked farro

1 cup chopped tomatoes

2 tablespoons chopped fresh parsley

Sea salt

Freshly ground black pepper

¼ cup shredded Parmesan cheese

1. Preheat the oven to 375°F.

2. Lightly grease a shallow 9-by-13-inch baking dish with oil.

3. Cut the tops off the bell peppers and take out the seeds. Place the peppers in the baking dish and set aside.

4. Heat the oil in a large skillet over medium-high heat, and sauté the beef until cooked through, about 8 minutes.

5. Add the onion, carrot, and garlic and sauté 4 minutes more.

6. Remove from the heat and stir in the spinach, farro, tomatoes, and parsley. Season the filling with salt and pepper.

7. Spoon the beef mixture into the peppers and sprinkle with the Parmesan.

8. Bake until the peppers are tender and the filling is completely heated through, 40 to 45 minutes.

Make Ahead: Cook the farro using 1 cup of grains and 2½ cups of water. Simmer for 30 to 40 minutes, until tender.

PER SERVING: Calories: 278; Total fat: 10g; Saturated fat: 3g; Sodium: 140mg; Carbohydrates: 19g; Fiber: 5g; Protein: 18g

Roasted Pork Chops with Chickpea–Cherry Tomato Salsa

SERVES 4 / PREP TIME: 10 MINUTES / COOK TIME: 18 MINUTES

5 INGREDIENTS OR LESS, 30 MINUTES OR LESS, ALLERGEN-FREE, DAIRY-FREE, NUT-FREE, ONE POT, UNDER 500 CALORIES

Although the recommended salsa is a gorgeous, healthy topping, any salsa is delicious with tender, roasted pork chops. Center-cut chops are lean and have very little visible fat. They are high in protein, which is a recommended nutrient for weight loss. Proteins can help you feel fuller longer, especially when combined with a complex carbohydrate such as salsa or a grain side dish.

4 (4-ounce) center-cut pork chops, trimmed of fat

1 teaspoon dried thyme

Sea salt

Freshly ground black pepper

1 tablespoon olive oil

1 cup Chickpea–Cherry Tomato Salsa (page 168), room temperature

1. Preheat the oven to 375°F.

2. Rub the pork chops all over with thyme, and lightly season with salt and pepper.

3. Heat the oil in a large oven-safe skillet over medium-high heat.

4. Brown the pork chops on all sides, about 8 minutes.

5. Place the skillet in the oven, and roast until the pork is just cooked through, about 10 minutes.

6. Serve with the salsa.

Variation Tip: You can make the pork chops on a grill with excellent results. Grilling is a great low-fat method of cooking meats, and it adds a pleasing, lightly charred taste that goes well with the slightly sweet fresh salsa.

PER SERVING: Calories: 293; Total fat: 17g; Saturated fat: 6g; Sodium: 253mg; Carbohydrates: 11g; Fiber: 2g; Protein: 22g

Broccoli-Beef Stir-Fry with Black Bean Sauce

SERVES 4 / PREP TIME: 15 MINUTES / COOK TIME: 22 MINUTES

DAIRY-FREE, UNDER 500 CALORIES

You might recognize this dish from your favorite Chinese restaurant; the combination of beef, broccoli, and black bean sauce is very popular. Here, toasty chopped cashews add crunch and healthy fat. Cashews, an excellent source of healthy oleic acid, are the seed of the cashew apple and not a nut at all, although it is classified as a tree nut for those with allergies.

1 tablespoon sesame oil

12 ounces beef sirloin, thinly sliced

1 head broccoli, separated into small florets

1 red bell pepper, thinly sliced

3 tablespoons store-bought black bean sauce

½ cup low-sodium beef broth

1 tablespoon cornstarch

2 scallions, white and green parts, thinly sliced on a bias

¼ cup chopped cashews

1. Heat the oil a large skillet or wok over medium-high heat.

2. Add the beef and sauté until just cooked through and lightly browned, about 8 minutes. Remove the beef to a plate with a slotted spoon, cover with foil, and set aside.

3. Add the broccoli and bell pepper to the skillet, and sauté until the broccoli is tender, about 7 minutes.

4. Add the black bean sauce and reserved beef, and sauté for 3 minutes.

5. In a small bowl, stir together the broth and cornstarch, add it to the skillet, and cook until the sauce thickens, about 4 minutes.

6. Serve topped with scallions and cashews.

Variation Tip: You can make your own bean sauce by bringing to a boil 2 cups of canned black beans, 1 tablespoon of low-sodium soy sauce, 1 teaspoon of orange zest, 1 teaspoon of grated fresh ginger, and 1 teaspoon of minced garlic in a small saucepan. Then reduce the heat to low and simmer for 25 minutes. You can add a pinch of red pepper flakes for some heat as well.

PER SERVING: Calories: 305; Total fat: 12g; Saturated fat: 1g; Sodium: 372mg; Carbohydrates: 25g; Fiber: 6g; Protein: 27g

Pork–Bok Choy Chow Mein

SERVES 4 / PREP TIME: 20 MINUTES / COOK TIME: 20 MINUTES

DAIRY-FREE, NUT-FREE, UNDER 500 CALORIES

Tender noodles, tasty pork, heaps of colorful vegetables, and a delicious light sauce combine to create the perfect dish to serve special guests—or keep all for yourself, because it is addictive. The toasted sesame oil lifts the other ingredients to a sublime culinary level, and the scent will delight your senses. Sesame oil is a rich source of monounsaturated and polyunsaturated fats, so this oil can decrease the risk of type 2 diabetes, dementia, and cardiovascular disease.

6 ounces dry chow mein noodles

3 teaspoons sesame oil, divided

½ pound lean ground pork

2 teaspoons minced garlic

2 teaspoons peeled grated fresh ginger

2 tablespoons low-sodium tamari sauce

1 tablespoon oyster sauce

2 cups shredded bok choy

2 celery stalks, thinly sliced

1 cup shredded carrot

2 scallions, white and green parts, thinly sliced

1 tablespoon sesame seeds, for garnish

1. Place a medium saucepan filled three-quarters with water over high heat, and bring to a boil.

2. Cook the noodles until tender, about 2 minutes, drain, and toss with 1 teaspoon of oil to prevent sticking. Set aside.

3. Heat the remaining 2 teaspoons of oil in a large skillet over medium-high heat.

4. Sauté the pork until just cooked through, about 7 minutes.

5. Stir in the garlic, ginger, tamari sauce, and oyster sauce, and cook until the ginger and garlic are softened, about 3 minutes.

6. Add the bok choy, celery, carrot, and scallions, and stir until the vegetables are tender, 7 to 8 minutes.

7. Stir in the noodles and toss to combine.

8. Serve topped with sesame seeds.

Substitution Tip: Omit the pork to create a vegan meal, or try beef or lean chicken breast for tasty variations.

PER SERVING: Calories: 322; Total fat: 14g; Saturated fat: 4g; Sodium: 543mg; Carbohydrates: 33g; Fiber: 5g; Protein: 18g

Kale-Beef Rolls

SERVES 4 / PREP TIME: 25 MINUTES / COOK TIME: 35 MINUTES

ALLERGEN-FREE, DAIRY-FREE, NUT-FREE, UNDER 500 CALORIES

If you have ever made cabbage rolls, you will find this preparation quite familiar, even if the ingredients are a little different. Cabbage rolls feature rice, whereas this version uses cooked quinoa. More than 5,000 years ago, quinoa was a staple in the Incan culture and was considered to be a sacred ingredient. Not only did they eat quinoa, but they also washed their clothes with the water used to rinse the soapy saponin coating off it. Quinoa is a seed, not a grain, and is very high in protein and fiber. It is a perfect complement for the beef and hearty kale wrapping of this tomato-baked dish.

12 medium kale leaves, hard stems removed

1 tablespoon olive oil, plus extra for greasing

12 ounces extra-lean ground beef

1 sweet onion, chopped

1 tablespoon minced garlic

2 teaspoons sweet paprika

1 teaspoon dried oregano

1 cup cooked quinoa

Sea salt

Freshly ground black pepper

1 (28-ounce) can low-sodium crushed tomatoes

¼ cup low-sodium beef broth

1 tablespoon chopped fresh parsley

1. Preheat the oven to 450°F. Lightly grease a 9-by-13-inch baking dish with oil and set aside.

2. Put a large saucepan filled three-quarters with water on high heat and bring to a boil.

3. Blanch the kale leaves (put the leaves in the boiling water until tender, drain and run the leaves under cold water, and pat them dry with paper towels) and set aside.

4. Heat the oil in a large skillet over medium-high heat.

5. Cook the beef until it is completely browned, about 7 minutes,

6. Stir in the onion, garlic, paprika, and oregano, and sauté until the vegetables are softened, about 3 minutes more.

CONTINUED >

7. Stir the quinoa into the meat mixture and season with salt and pepper.

8. Spread a quarter of the crushed tomatoes into the baking dish.

9. Lay out one of the kale leaves and spoon the filling into the center. Tuck in the sides of the leaf and roll it up tightly. Place the roll seam-side down in the baking pan.

10. Repeat with the remaining leaves and filling.

11. Pour the rest of the crushed tomatoes and the broth over the kale rolls.

12. Bake until the sauce is bubbling, and the kale rolls are completely heated through, about 20 minutes.

13. Serve topped with parsley.

Make Ahead: Throw together a couple of pans of this hearty casserole to bake straight from the freezer when you want an effortless meal. Cover the frozen casserole with aluminum foil for the first 45 minutes of baking in a 375°F oven, then uncover and bake another 15 minutes.

PER SERVING: Calories: 361; Total fat: 11g; Saturated fat: 3g; Sodium: 247mg; Carbohydrates: 40g; Fiber: 6g; Protein: 25g

Rustic Beef & Cabbage Stew

SERVES 4 / PREP TIME: 15 MINUTES / COOK TIME: 41 MINUTES

ALLERGEN-FREE, DAIRY-FREE, NUT-FREE, ONE POT, UNDER 500 CALORIES

Stew is the ultimate comfort food; it fills you up and seems to warm your body right down to your toes on a chilly winter day. Cabbage provides the majority of the bulk in this stew, along with lean ground beef and pale navy beans. Cabbage is a crucial ingredient for lowering cholesterol because it binds with bile acids in your digestive system and helps remove them from the body. Reduced bile acids equal less cholesterol and a healthier cardiovascular system.

1 tablespoon olive oil

12 ounces extra-lean ground beef

1 sweet onion, chopped

1 tablespoon minced garlic

1 (28-ounce) can low-sodium stewed tomatoes

1 (15-ounce) low-sodium navy beans, drained and rinsed

3 cups shredded cabbage

1 cup low-sodium beef broth

2 carrots, sliced

1 large parsnip, thinly sliced

2 teaspoons chopped fresh thyme

Sea salt

Freshly ground black pepper

1. Heat the oil in a large saucepan over medium-high heat.

2. Sauté the ground beef until cooked through, about 8 minutes.

3. Stir in the onion and garlic and cook until softened, about 3 minutes.

4. Stir in the tomatoes, navy beans, cabbage, broth, carrots, parsnip, and thyme and simmer until the vegetables are tender, about 30 minutes.

5. Season with salt and pepper and serve.

Make Ahead: Double this recipe and freeze it for up to 2 months in handy one-cup servings for a quick meal. Thaw the stew in the refrigerator overnight and reheat on the stove or in the microwave.

PER SERVING: Calories: 370; Total fat: 10g; Saturated fat: 3g; Sodium: 376mg; Carbohydrates: 46g; Fiber: 14g; Protein: 26g

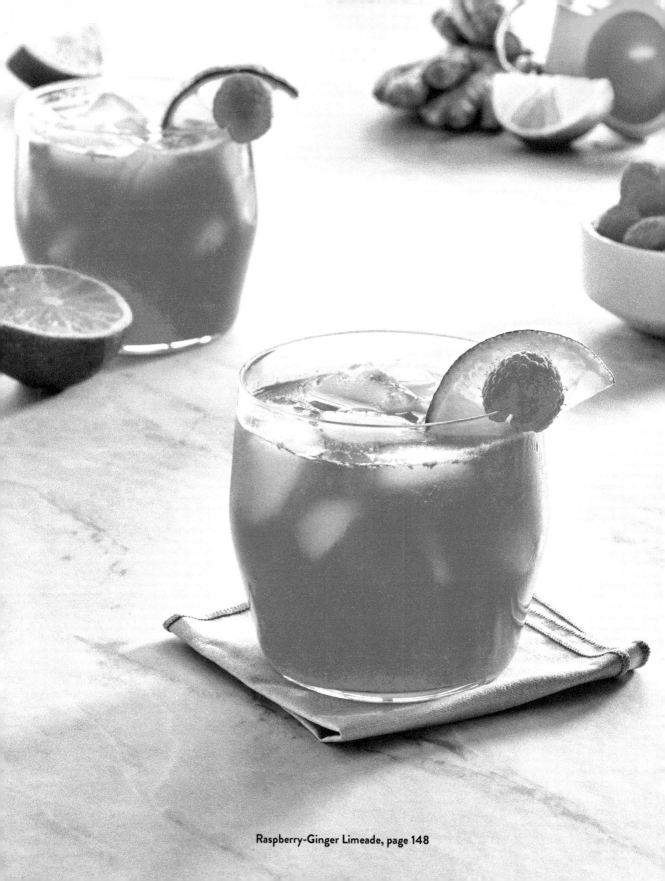

Raspberry-Ginger Limeade, page 148

CHAPTER 10

SMALL MEALS & FAST-FRIENDLY BEVERAGES

Quenching Cucumber-Lime Juice

SERVES 2 / PREP TIME: 10 MINUTES

30 MINUTES OR LESS, ALLERGEN-FREE, DAIRY-FREE, NUT-FREE, ONE POT, UNDER 500 CALORIES, VEGAN

Cucumber is an underrated vegetable; it's incredibly refreshing and very nutritious. It is low calorie and very high in water and soluble fiber, so it can be a terrific choice for weight loss. Cucumber is an excellent source of beta-carotene; vitamins A, C, and K; as well as potassium and magnesium. Try this tart juice as a diuretic that can also reduce inflammation and blood pressure.

2 cups water

1 English cucumber, sliced

2 limes, peeled

1 tablespoon apple cider vinegar

1 teaspoon chopped fresh mint

1. Place the water, cucumber, limes, vinegar, and mint in a blender and pulse until very smooth.

2. Pour into glasses and serve immediately.

Craving Tip: You should be drinking lots of water when fasting, and this juice is a nice stand-in when your taste buds need a bit of flavor. Incredibly fresh-tasting with a hint of sweet and sour, this juice should be enjoyed before eating your main meal.

PER SERVING: Calories: 15; Total fat: 0g; Saturated fat: 0g; Sodium: 5mg; Carbohydrates: 4g; Fiber: 3g; Protein: 2g

Basic Vegetable Broth

MAKES 8 CUPS / PREP TIME: 15 MINUTES / COOK TIME: 2 TO 3 HOURS

ALLERGEN-FREE, DAIRY-FREE, NUT-FREE, UNDER 500 CALORIES

The flavor of homemade broth is dependent on the types of herbs and vegetables you simmer together, so make sure your ingredients aren't just scraps. You can certainly throw in carrot tops, onion ends, and the stems from herbs used in other recipes, but you might not like the finished flavor. Parsley is a nice choice because it adds a fresh taste and contains flavonoids that make their way into the broth. These flavonoids can help prevent cell damage, especially to blood vessels.

5 garlic cloves, crushed

4 celery stalks with leaves, roughly chopped

2 carrots, roughly chopped

1 onion, quartered

½ cup chopped fresh parsley

3 thyme sprigs

2 bay leaves

½ teaspoon black peppercorns

¼ teaspoon salt

8 cups water

1. In a large stockpot, place the garlic, celery, carrots, onion, parsley, thyme, bay leaves, and peppercorns.

2. Add the water, cover, and bring to a boil.

3. Reduce the heat to low and gently simmer for 2 to 3 hours.

4. Strain the broth through a fine-mesh sieve and discard the solids.

5. Refrigerate broth in sealed containers for up to 5 days or freeze for up to 1 month.

PER (1-CUP) SERVING: Calories: 24; Total fat: 0g; Total carbohydrates: 4g; Net carbs: 4g; Fiber: 0g; Protein: 2g

Beef Broth Variation: Add 2 to 3 pounds of beef bones (beef marrow, knuckle bones, ribs, and any other bones) and 2 tablespoons of apple cider vinegar to the basic broth recipe along with enough water to

CONTINUED >

cover the extra ingredients. Simmer, scooping off any accumulating foam, for 6 to 7 hours. Strain the broth through a fine-mesh sieve, discarding the solids. Store cooled broth in sealed containers in the refrigerator for up to 1 week or in the freezer for up to 3 months.

PER (1-CUP) SERVING: Calories: 42; Total fat: 1g; Total carbohydrates: 0g; Net carbs: 0g; Fiber: 0g; Protein: 8g

Chicken Broth Variation: Add 2 whole chickens and 2 tablespoons of apple cider vinegar to the basic broth recipe along with enough water to cover the extra ingredients. Simmer, scooping off any accumulating foam, for 4 to 5 hours. Strain the broth through a fine-mesh sieve, discarding the solids. Store cooled broth in sealed containers in the refrigerator for up to 1 week or in the freezer for up to 3 months.

PER (1-CUP) SERVING: Calories: 38; Total fat: 0g; Total carbohydrates: 0g; Net carbs: 0g; Fiber: 0g; Protein: 9g

Fish Broth Variation: Add 3 to 4 pounds of fish heads and bones to the basic broth recipe along with enough water to cover the extra ingredients. Simmer (do not boil) for 1 hour, then strain through a fine-mesh sieve, discarding the solids. Store cooled broth in sealed containers in the refrigerator for up to 1 week or in the freezer for up to 3 months.

PER (1-CUP) SERVING: Calories: 34; Total fat: 1g; Total carbohydrates: 0g; Net carbs: 0g; Fiber: 0g; Protein: 7g

Peppermint-Mocha Coffee

SERVES 1 / PREP TIME: 5 MINUTES

Mocha means a blend of coffee and chocolate; what could be better than that to start your day? This recipe uses a generous portion of cocoa powder, so the chocolate flavor is quite distinct. If you want a more subtle flavor, reduce the amount to 1 or 2 teaspoons. Cocoa is a traditional folk remedy that may help reduce the risk of diabetes and protect against cardiovascular disease.

1 cup freshly
brewed coffee

¼ cup skim milk or
unsweetened
almond milk

1 tablespoon
cocoa powder

1 teaspoon maple syrup
(optional)

2 drops pure
peppermint extract

1. Place the coffee, milk, cocoa powder, maple syrup (if using), and peppermint extract in a blender and pulse until frothy, about 30 seconds.

2. Pour the coffee into a large mug and serve.

Variation Tip: This recipe is also delicious served cold over ice if you prefer a chilled beverage. Triple the recipe and store it in a pitcher in the refrigerator to enjoy at your convenience.

PER SERVING: Calories: 34; Total fat: 1g; Saturated fat: 0g; Sodium: 34mg; Carbohydrates: 6g; Fiber: 2g; Protein: 3g

Green Energy Juice

SERVES 4 / PREP TIME: 5 MINUTES

5 INGREDIENTS OR LESS, 30 MINUTES OR LESS, NUT-FREE, ONE POT,
UNDER 500 CALORIES, VEGAN

Celery adds a slightly salty flavor to this nutrient-packed beverage, especially if you keep the frothy greens on the stalks or use the inner stalks. Celery leaves have five times the amount of magnesium and calcium as the stalks—and they taste delicious, too. The leaves are also very high in immune-boosting vitamin C, so cut them off your celery bunch and store them in a plastic bag in the refrigerator for up to 1 week for other recipes.

3 cups water

¾ cup baby kale

½ English cucumber, cut into 1-inch chunks

2 celery stalks, plus greens, cut into 1-inch chunks

1 pear, cored

Juice of 1 lime

¼ cup fresh basil

Pinch ground nutmeg

1. Place the water, kale, cucumber, celery, pear, lime juice, basil, and nutmeg in a blender and pulse until liquified or very well blended.

2. Pour into a glass and serve immediately.

Variation Tip: You can prepare this recipe using a juicer instead of a blender if you want a more classic preparation. It will produce less volume and you will lose the fiber of the blended variation, but fresh juices can be beneficial in a fasting diet.

PER SERVING: Calories: 36; Total fat: 0g;
Saturated fat: 0g; Sodium: 11mg; Carbohydrates: 9g;
Fiber: 2g; Protein: 1g

Green Tea–Lemonade

SERVES 2 / PREP TIME: 10 MINUTES

5 INGREDIENTS OR LESS, 30 MINUTES OR LESS, DAIRY-FREE, NUT-FREE, ONE POT, UNDER 500 CALORIES, VEGAN

Green tea is often recommended for weight loss and is the main ingredient in many over-the-counter aids. Getting green tea in its liquid form is a fabulous way to access this beverage's many antioxidants such as catechins, specifically epigallocatechin gallate (EGCG), a metabolism booster. When EGCG is combined with the caffeine in the tea, you have a perfect mixture to accelerate fat loss.

2 cups cold-brewed green tea
Juice of 2 lemons
1 tablespoon honey
1 teaspoon peeled grated fresh ginger
½ teaspoon finely chopped fresh mint

1. In a medium pitcher, stir together the tea, lemon juice, honey, ginger, and mint.

2. Serve over ice.

Make Ahead: Cold-brewed tea makes an excellent addition to smoothies and other beverages such as this one, so make a pitcher ahead of time and store it in the refrigerator for your recipe needs. Different types of tea would be delicious in this recipe, such as peppermint, ginseng, and Earl Grey.

PER SERVING: Calories: 43; Total fat: 0g; Saturated fat: 0g; Sodium: 10mg; Carbohydrates: 8g; Fiber: 0g; Protein: 1g

Raspberry-Ginger Limeade

SERVES 4 / PREP TIME: 10 MINUTES

The most prominent flavor in this pretty pink beverage is ginger, giving it a touch of heat and potent healing properties. Ginger is a medicinal ingredient used for gastric problems, including nausea, and for relieving arthritis pain. Look for plump ginger rhizomes with no wizened ends or soft spots. Ginger will keep in the vegetable crisper of your refrigerator for up to 2 weeks.

2 cups fresh raspberries
½ cup freshly squeezed lime juice
2 tablespoons honey
2 tablespoons peeled grated fresh ginger
6 cups water

1. Place the raspberries, lime juice, honey, and ginger into a blender and pulse until very well blended.

2. Strain the liquid through a fine-mesh sieve into a pitcher to remove the seeds and pulp.

3. Pour in the water and serve.

4. Store extra limeade in the refrigerator for up to 4 days.

Variation Tip: Any type of fruit can be used in this lovely beverage, such as strawberries, peaches, cherries, or tropical mango. If you use a seedless fruit, you can skip the second step.

PER SERVING: Calories: 80; Total fat: 1g; Saturated fat: 0g; Sodium: 14mg; Carbohydrates: 16g; Fiber: 4g; Protein: 1g

Gingerbread Breakfast Bars

MAKES 16 BARS / PREP TIME: 10 MINUTES / COOK TIME: 20 MINUTES

30 MINUTES OR LESS, DAIRY-FREE, UNDER 500 CALORIES, VEGAN

Granola bars are often a grab-and-go breakfast or meal for the chronically time-starved, but store-bought bars are not usually a healthy choice due to their high sugar and saturated fat content. Homemade bars allow you to control the ingredients and tailor the recipe to your own taste. Pecans add a lovely buttery flavor, and the healthy fats in the nuts are one of the binders to keep the bars together. If you omit them, be sure to replace them with another nut for texture and structure purposes.

2 cups rolled oats

1 cup almond flour

½ cup chopped pecans

2 teaspoons ground ginger

1 teaspoon ground cinnamon

¼ teaspoon baking soda

½ cup unsweetened applesauce

¼ cup maple syrup

2 tablespoons molasses

1 teaspoon pure vanilla extract

1. Preheat the oven to 350°F. Line a 9-by-13-inch baking dish with parchment paper and set aside.

2. In a large bowl, mix together the oats, almond flour, pecans, ginger, cinnamon, and baking soda until well blended.

3. In a small bowl, stir together the applesauce, maple syrup, molasses, and vanilla.

4. Add the wet ingredients to the dry ingredients and stir until mixed well.

5. Transfer the mixture to the baking dish and press it down firmly in an even layer.

6. Bake the mixture until lightly golden, about 20 minutes.

CONTINUED >

7. Allow to cool for 20 minutes, then cut into 16 bars.

8. Cool completely before removing them from the pan.

9. Store the breakfast bars in a sealed container in the refrigerator for up to 1 week.

Variation Tip: Mashed banana can take the place of the applesauce if you want a sweeter bar without adding more maple syrup. The banana can be added in the same amount, and you might enjoy the slightly dense texture of the bars.

PER SERVING (1 BAR): Calories: 107; Total fat: 5g; Saturated fat:1g; Sodium: 23mg; Carbohydrates: 14g; Fiber: 2g; Protein: 3g

Bulgur Lettuce Tacos

SERVES 4 / PREP TIME: 25 MINUTES

30 MINUTES OR LESS, ALLERGEN-FREE, DAIRY-FREE, NUT-FREE, ONE POT,
UNDER 500 CALORIES, VEGAN

Lettuce wraps don't have to be spicy and filled with meats or fish; they can be a simple, wholesome meal of grains, vegetables, and seeds. The sunflower seed topping adds a lovely crunch and nutty finish and is an ideal choice for weight loss and a heart-friendly diet. The seeds are packed with polyunsaturated fats, protein, fiber, and vitamin E, and also contain copper and folate.

1 cup cooked bulgur

1 large tomato, chopped

1 English cucumber, chopped

1 red bell pepper, chopped

½ cup shredded carrot

¼ red onion, chopped

2 tablespoons freshly squeezed lemon juice

1 tablespoon olive oil

Sea salt

Freshly ground black pepper

8 large Boston lettuce leaves

¼ cup roasted unsalted sunflower seeds

1. In a large bowl, mix together the bulgur, tomato, cucumber, bell pepper, carrot, onion, lemon juice, and oil.

2. Season with salt and pepper.

3. Scoop the bulgur mixture into each lettuce leaf and fold like a taco.

4. Top with the sunflower seeds and serve.

Make Ahead: The bulgur can be made ahead (see tip page 108), or you can use canned navy beans or black beans instead in a pinch. The grain adds a lovely texture and slightly nutty flavor, so it is the first choice.

PER SERVING: Calories: 136; Total fat: 6g;
Saturated fat: 1g; Sodium: 79mg; Carbohydrates: 19g;
Fiber: 5g; Protein: 5g

Baked Egg & Herb Portobello Mushrooms

SERVES 4 / PREP TIME: 15 MINUTES / COOK TIME: 10 MINUTES

5 INGREDIENTS OR LESS, 30 MINUTES OR LESS, DAIRY-FREE, NUT-FREE, UNDER 500 CALORIES, VEGAN

Portobello mushrooms are often used in place of meat because they have a firm texture and hold up well in most cooking applications. In this recipe, perfectly sunny-side up eggs are baked with fragrant thyme right in the mushrooms—tasty and beautiful. Mushrooms are a good source of fiber and protein and are the only plant source of vitamin D. The antioxidants found in mushrooms can help fight cancer and boost the immune system. Always buy loose mushrooms rather than packaged so that you can check that they are not wet, slimy, or shriveled.

4 large portobello mushrooms, stemmed with black gills scooped out
2 tablespoons olive oil
1 teaspoon chopped fresh thyme
4 large eggs
Sea salt
Freshly ground black pepper
1 teaspoon chopped fresh chives, for garnish

1. Preheat the oven to broil.

2. Place the mushrooms hollow-side down on a baking sheet and broil until tender, about 3 minutes.

3. Flip the mushrooms, drizzle the oil on them, sprinkle with the thyme, and broil 3 minutes more.

4. Remove the baking sheet from the oven, and carefully crack the eggs into the mushrooms, one per mushroom.

5. Broil the mushrooms until the egg whites are cooked through, 3 to 4 minutes.

6. Season the mushrooms with salt and pepper, sprinkle with chives, and serve.

Variation Tip: This recipe can also be prepared on a barbecue on medium-high heat. Simply grill the mushrooms and follow the recipe as directed. Close the lid on your grill when cooking the eggs to contain the heat and cook the eggs well.

PER SERVING: Calories: 149; Total fat: 12g; Saturated fat: 3g; Sodium: 129mg; Carbohydrates: 6g; Fiber: 1g; Protein: 9g

Miso, Snow Pea & Tofu Soup

SERVES 2 / PREP TIME: 15 MINUTES / COOK TIME: 5 MINUTES

30 MINUTES OR LESS, DAIRY-FREE, NUT-FREE, UNDER 500 CALORIES, VEGAN

Miso is a familiar ingredient in many Japanese dishes, and even if you have not yet used this paste in your own recipes, the flavor might remind you of your favorite takeout. Miso—made from soybeans, grains, and salt—is salty, tangy, and slightly sweet. There are more than 1,000 types of miso, but you will probably see only one or two in your local grocery store, depending on where you live. The amino acids in miso support the immune system, and the enzymes and good bacteria can strengthen the digestive system, promoting weight loss and good health.

4 cups Basic Vegetable Broth (page 143) or low-sodium vegetable broth, divided

3 to 4 tablespoons miso paste

4 ounces silken tofu, cut into ½-inch cubes

½ cup snow peas, trimmed and cut into ½-inch pieces

½ red bell pepper, diced

¼ cup shredded carrot

1 scallion, white and green parts, thinly sliced diagonally on a bias

1. Heat 3½ cups of broth in a medium saucepan over medium-high heat and bring to a boil.

2. Reduce the heat to low so that the broth simmers gently.

3. In a small bowl, whisk together the remaining ½ cup of broth and the miso until smooth. Set aside.

4. Add the tofu, snow peas, bell pepper, and carrot to the simmering broth. Simmer until the tofu is heated through and the vegetables are tender, about 5 minutes.

5. Remove from the heat and stir in the miso mixture.

6. Serve topped with scallion.

Addition Tip: Serve this simple soup as an accompaniment to a larger meal such as Curried Peanut Vegetable Noodles (page 104) or Pork–Bok Choy Chow Mein (page 136). This will increase the calories to more than 400 and 500, respectively.

PER SERVING: Calories: 151; Total fat: 3g; Saturated fat: 1g; Sodium: 931mg; Carbohydrates: 17g; Fiber: 4g; Protein: 13g

Fruit & Nut Yogurt Parfait

SERVES 4 / PREP TIME: 15 MINUTES

30 MINUTES OR LESS, UNDER 500 CALORIES, VEGAN

Parfaits are lovely layers of fruit, creamy filling of some type (yogurt in this recipe), and crunchy nuts or seeds. The fruit in this version is just a suggestion, but strawberries are always a delicious choice. They are sweet enough not to need any artificial enhancement and contain many health benefits: they can support eye health, lower cholesterol, and support the immune system as well as reduce the risk of chronic diseases such as diabetes and heart disease.

¼ cup roasted unsalted
   pumpkin seeds
2 tablespoons
   chopped pecans
2 tablespoons
   hemp hearts
½ cup raspberries
½ cup sliced strawberries
½ cup halved, pitted black
   cherries
½ cup diced peach or
   nectarine
8 ounces plain
   Greek yogurt

1. In a small bowl, stir together the pumpkin seeds, pecans, and hemp hearts.

2. In a small bowl, toss together the raspberries, strawberries, cherries, and peach.

3. Scoop one-quarter cup of the fruit into the bottom of 4 glasses, top each with 1 ounce of yogurt, then 1 tablespoon of the seed mixture. Repeat with the remaining fruit, yogurt, and seed mixture to create pretty layers.

4. Serve immediately or store in the refrigerator for up to 4 hours.

Addition Tip: Serve this parfait as a pairing with Baked Cinnamon-Orange French Toast (page 76) or Ricotta-Oatmeal Pancakes (page 79) for an attractive and filling breakfast. You can also double up on the portion size of the parfait to create a 300-calorie meal.

PER SERVING: Calories: 153; Total fat: 7g; Saturated fat: 1g; Sodium: 36mg; Carbohydrates: 13g; Fiber: 3g; Protein: 12g

Rich Butter Coffee

SERVES 1 / PREP TIME: 1 MINUTE

5 INGREDIENTS OR LESS, 30 MINUTES OR LESS, NUT-FREE,
UNDER 500 CALORIES, VEGAN

Butter and coffee seem like a crazy combination unless you have kept up with the keto and low-carb diets that are currently trending. When you blend this popular beverage with the fats, culinary magic seems to happen. The resulting drink is creamy and frothy and has a lovely, lightly salty and nutty taste. You might think the added fat is not conducive to weight loss, but the butter and oil actually increase the feeling of fullness and slow digestion; you will not feel hungry and will eat less.

1 cup freshly brewed black coffee
1 tablespoon butter
½ tablespoon coconut oil

1. Place the coffee, butter, and oil in a blender and pulse until creamy, about 30 seconds.

2. Serve immediately.

Addition Tip: Top this luscious beverage with a generous scoop of whipped cream or whipped coconut cream for a coffeehouse experience. This addition will add 75 calories and 30 calories, respectively.

PER SERVING: Calories: 160; Total fat: 18g; Saturated fat: 13g; Sodium: 82mg; Carbohydrates: 0g; Fiber: 0g; Protein: 0g

Fresh Green Bean Salad with Herbs

SERVES 4 / PREP TIME: 15 MINUTES / COOK TIME: 3 MINUTES

30 MINUTES OR LESS, ALLERGEN-FREE, DAIRY-FREE, NUT-FREE, UNDER 500 CALORIES, VEGAN

Bean salad is a staple dish in potlucks and family gatherings because it is simple to prepare and the flavor is pleasant and familiar to most people. Three types of beans grace this recipe: fresh snap beans and two kinds of legumes. Navy beans are a very mild bean, with a buttery texture and a lot of fiber, which can stabilize blood sugar while lowering cholesterol. Make sure you rinse the canned beans even if they are low in sodium to remove any additives or excess salt from them.

6 cups fresh green beans, cut into 1-inch pieces
½ cup low-sodium canned navy beans, drained and rinsed
½ cup low-sodium canned lentils, drained and rinsed
1 tablespoon chopped fresh basil
¼ cup Oil & Vinegar Dressing (page 170)
Sea salt
Freshly ground black pepper

1. Place a large pot three-quarters full of water on high heat and bring to a boil.

2. Add the beans and blanch until just tender, about 3 minutes.

3. Drain the beans and run them under cold water.

4. Pat the beans dry with a clean kitchen towel and transfer them to a large bowl.

5. Stir in the navy beans, lentils, basil, and dressing, tossing to coat.

6. Season the salad with salt and pepper and serve.

Make Ahead: Bean salads get better and better as they sit and "pickle" in the dressing. This salad can be made a day ahead and stored in the refrigerator in a sealed container to mellow and deepen the flavors.

PER SERVING: Calories: 184; Total fat: 9g; Saturated fat: 1g; Sodium: 31mg; Carbohydrates: 23g; Fiber: 10g; Protein: 7g

Chicken & Artichoke Heart Pita Pizzas

SERVES 4 / PREP TIME: 15 MINUTES / COOK TIME: 20 MINUTES

ONE POT, NUT-FREE, UNDER 500 CALORIES

Pizza is a favorite meal for many because every taste can be satisfied depending on the sauce, toppings, and cheese. Artichoke hearts are a fancier topping, adding texture and a tangy flavor to the dish. Artichokes can be eaten fresh, frozen, or as the marinated ingredient found here. Artichoke hearts are packed with antioxidants that can protect against heart disease and provide filling fiber. Make sure you purchase artichoke hearts that are not packed in oil so the calorie count remains low.

2 (6-inch) whole-wheat pita breads

1 teaspoon olive oil

2 tomatoes, thinly sliced

½ cup chopped cooked chicken breasts

½ cup chopped marinated artichoke hearts

½ cup blanched chopped spinach, liquid squeezed out

¼ cup shredded Parmesan cheese

1 tablespoon chopped fresh basil

1. Preheat the oven to 400°F.

2. Put the pitas on a baking sheet and brush them with the oil.

3. Place the pitas in the oven and bake until lightly browned, about 5 minutes.

4. Remove the sheet from the oven and arrange the tomato slices on the pitas.

5. Evenly divide the chicken breast, artichoke hearts, spinach, and Parmesan between the pitas, scattering the ingredients across the whole surface of each pita.

6. Bake the pizzas in the oven until the bread is golden and crispy and the toppings heated through, 10 to 15 minutes. Serve.

Craving Tip: Sometimes, a decadent treat is what you need to satisfy your craving for "junk" food. This isn't a fat-drenched high-calorie store-bought pizza, but it is more than satisfying.

PER SERVING: Calories: 193; Total fat: 7g; Saturated fat: 2g; Sodium: 280mg; Carbohydrates: 21g; Fiber: 5g; Protein: 11g

Classic Eggs & Canadian Bacon

SERVES 2 / PREP TIME: 2 MINUTES / COOK TIME: 8 MINUTES

5 INGREDIENTS OR LESS, 30 MINUTES OR LESS, DAIRY-FREE, NUT-FREE, UNDER 500 CALORIES

Bacon and eggs can be part of a weight-loss plan if you use Canadian bacon instead of the standard smoked pork belly. Canadian bacon (aka peameal bacon, known as back bacon in Canada) is made from the lean loin of the animal and is cured like ham, so it is lower in fat and calories. You can slice your own from a bigger piece or buy this delicious meat presliced to ensure portion size.

3 teaspoons olive oil, divided

4 ounces Canadian bacon, cut into ¼-inch slices

2 large eggs

Sea salt

Freshly ground black pepper

1 large tomato, sliced

1. Heat 2 teaspoons of oil in a large skillet over medium-high heat.

2. Cook the bacon until it is lightly golden on both sides, about 6 minutes, flipping once.

3. Remove the bacon to a plate and cover it with aluminum foil to keep it warm.

4. Reduce the heat to medium, add the remaining 1 teaspoon of oil to the skillet, and crack in the eggs.

5. Let the eggs fry, tilting the pan occasionally to redistribute the uncooked whites until the edges are slightly crisp and the yolk is cooked, about 2 minutes for runny yolks or 3 minutes for medium-firm yolks.

6. Season the eggs with salt and pepper. To serve, place 1 egg, 2 pieces of Canadian bacon, and 2 tomato slices on each plate.

Substitution Tip: Use lean ham or slices of grilled or broiled sweet potato instead of the Canadian bacon for a different taste profile. The ham is lower in calories, and the sweet potato creates a vegetarian option.

PER SERVING: Calories: 199; Total fat: 13g; Saturated fat: 4g; Sodium: 389mg; Carbohydrates: 6g; Fiber: 2g; Protein: 18g

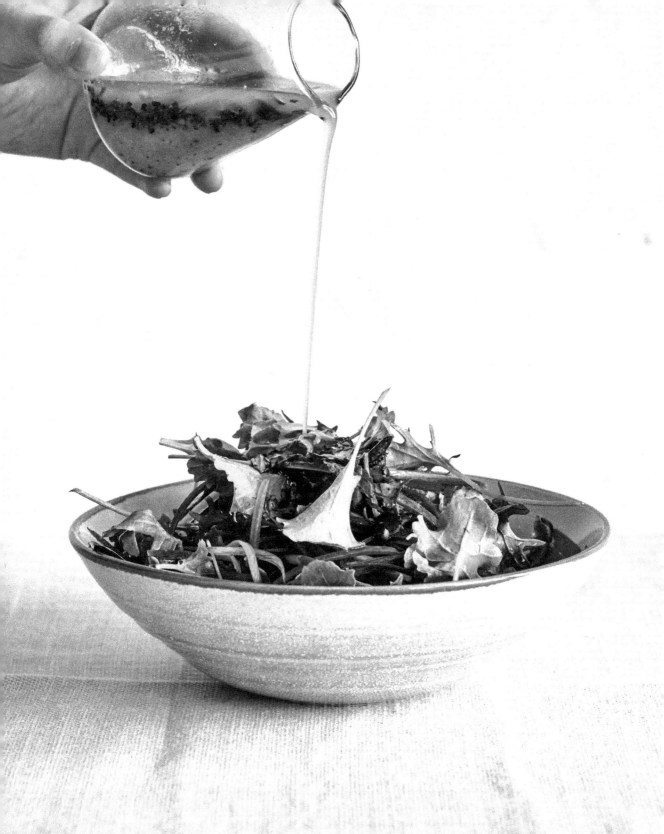

Orange-Cilantro Vinaigrette, page 169

CHAPTER 11

CONDIMENTS, SAUCES & DRESSINGS

Maple Barbecue Sauce

MAKES 1 CUP / PREP TIME: 10 MINUTES / COOK TIME: 15 MINUTES

30 MINUTES OR LESS, ALLERGEN-FREE, DAIRY-FREE, NUT-FREE, ONE POT, UNDER 500 CALORIES, VEGAN

A staple barbecue sauce is a must-have in your culinary repertoire, because it can quickly transform a simple grilled or broiled protein into a tempting meal. Balsamic vinegar and maple syrup add a pleasing sweetness to this slightly hot sauce. If you are not a fan of heat, omit the red pepper flakes and Dijon mustard.

½ cup unsalted
  tomato paste
¼ cup water
1 tablespoon balsamic
  vinegar
1 tablespoon maple syrup
1 tablespoon
  Worcestershire sauce
1 tablespoon
  Dijon mustard
1 teaspoon minced garlic
1 shallot, minced
½ teaspoon
  smoked paprika
¼ teaspoon red
  pepper flakes

1. In a small saucepan, whisk together the tomato paste, water, vinegar, maple syrup, Worcestershire sauce, mustard, garlic, shallot, paprika, and red pepper flakes until well blended.

2. Place the saucepan over medium heat and bring the mixture to a boil. Reduce the heat to low and simmer, stirring frequently until the sauce is thickened, about 15 minutes.

3. Cool completely and store in a sealed container in the refrigerator for up to 1 week.

Variation Tip: Try a teaspoon of liquid smoke for a truly spectacular barbecue sauce. You can find it in most grocery stores in the specialty food aisles or in a store specializing in grills or kitchen products.

PER SERVING (2 TABLESPOONS): Calories: 27; Total fat: 0g; Saturated fat: 0g; Sodium: 53mg; Carbohydrates: 6g; Fiber: 1g, Protein: 1g

Honeyed Buttermilk Dressing

MAKES 1 CUP / PREP TIME: 5 MINUTES

5 INGREDIENTS OR LESS, 30 MINUTES OR LESS, NUT-FREE, ONE POT,
UNDER 500 CALORIES, VEGAN

Buttermilk was a staple in kitchens of the past because this tangy liquid was left over after butter was churned from fresh milk. Buttermilk sounds fatty, but much of the fat is taken out, so just the rich flavor remains. Real buttermilk can still contain saturated fat, so look for a low-fat product in your local supermarket if you want a very low-calorie dressing.

½ cup buttermilk
¼ cup honey
3 tablespoons apple
  cider vinegar
1 tablespoon poppy seeds
Pinch ground nutmeg
Sea salt

1. In a small bowl, whisk together the buttermilk, honey, vinegar, poppy seeds, and nutmeg until well blended.

2. Season with salt and shake well before serving.

3. Store the dressing in the refrigerator in a sealed container for up to 2 weeks.

Craving Tip: This dressing is luscious and adds an incredible richness to whatever salad or dish you add it to or drizzle it over. This subtle sweetness and tartness are satisfying, and the crunch of poppy seeds is a nice added texture.

PER SERVING (2 TABLESPOONS): Calories: 46;
Total fat: 1g; Saturated fat: 0g; Sodium: 48mg;
Carbohydrates: 10g; Fiber: 0g; Protein: 1g

Curried Peanut Sauce

MAKES 1 CUP / PREP TIME: 10 MINUTES

30 MINUTES OR LESS, DAIRY-FREE, ONE POT, UNDER 500 CALORIES, VEGAN

Peanut sauce is a versatile sauce for dipping, tossing with noodles or other spiralized vegetables, or as a sauce for a tasty stir-fry. You can create different layers of heat depending on the type of curry you add to the mixture, from mild to mouth-scorching hot. You can actually leave out the curry altogether if this flavor is not your favorite.

¾ cup light coconut milk

¼ cup natural peanut butter

1 tablespoon curry powder

1 teaspoon honey

½ teaspoon minced garlic

¼ teaspoon peeled grated fresh ginger

Sea salt

1. In a small bowl, whisk together the coconut milk, peanut butter, curry powder, honey, garlic, and ginger until well combined.

2. Season with salt and serve.

3. Store in a sealed container in the refrigerator for up to 1 week.

Craving Tip: This sauce is sweet, savory, and has a little heat to satisfy any type of craving you might have. Try it on vegetables, tossed with noodles, or spooned over grilled chicken or pork tenderloin for a delectable meal.

PER SERVING (2 TABLESPOONS): Calories: 68; Total fat: 5g; Saturated fat: 2g; Sodium: 8mg; Carbohydrates: 4g; Fiber: 1g; Protein: 3g

Garlic-Oregano Yogurt Sauce

MAKES 1 CUP / PREP TIME: 10 MINUTES

5 INGREDIENTS OR LESS, 30 MINUTES OR LESS, NUT-FREE,
UNDER 500 CALORIES, VEGAN

Garlic is popular in both culinary and medicinal applications, and this allium was even administered to athletes in ancient Greece to enhance their performance in sports. Garlic is thought to treat many ailments and conditions often linked to the cardiovascular system and blood, specifically high cholesterol, heart disease, and atherosclerosis. Think of this revered history when preparing this delicious sauce.

¾ cup plain Greek yogurt
½ cup finely chopped
  fresh oregano
1 tablespoon
  minced garlic
1 teaspoon honey
Sea salt
Freshly ground
  black pepper

1. Place the yogurt, oregano, garlic, and honey in a blender and pulse until very smooth.

2. Season with salt and pepper and serve.

3. Store in a sealed container in the refrigerator for up to 1 week.

Substitution Tip: Use silken tofu instead of yogurt and omit the honey to make a vegan sauce. Then try it on blanched or roasted vegetables for a delicious side dish or main meal.

PER SERVING (¼ CUP): Calories: 70; Total fat: 1g; Saturated fat: 0g; Sodium: 86mg; Carbohydrates: 11g; Fiber: 4g; Protein: 8g

Simple Raw Marinara Sauce

SERVES 4 / PREP TIME: 15 MINUTES, PLUS SOAKING TIME

30 MINUTES OR LESS, ALLERGEN-FREE, DAIRY-FREE, NUT-FREE,
UNDER 500 CALORIES, VEGAN

You might be wondering what the benefit is of creating a sauce from sun-dried tomatoes instead of from canned diced tomatoes; it is all about the taste. Sun-dried tomatoes are more intensely flavored, and the raw preparation with fresh herbs is sublime. For the best results, look for dried tomatoes in bags or boxes, not ones packed in oil or marinated.

2 cups sun-dried tomatoes

2 cups low-sodium vegetable broth or water

2 tablespoons tomato paste

2 garlic cloves

1 tablespoon chopped fresh basil

1 tablespoon chopped fresh oregano

Sea salt

Freshly ground black pepper

1. Soak the tomatoes in the broth until rehydrated, about 4 hours or overnight.

2. Place the tomatoes, soaking liquid, tomato paste, garlic, basil, and oregano in a blender and pulse until the sauce is smooth and thick.

3. Season with salt and pepper and serve.

4. Store in a sealed container in the refrigerator for up to 1 week.

Addition Tip: Use this sauce with whole-grain noodles or vegetable noodles, or as a topping for chicken, fish, or pork. You can stir it into soups or stews for a flavor boost.

PER SERVING: Calories: 82; Total fat: 1g; Saturated fat: 0g; Sodium: 124mg; Carbohydrates: 18g; Fiber: 4g; Protein: 4g

Herbed Guacamole

SERVES 4 / PREP TIME: 10 MINUTES

30 MINUTES OR LESS, NUT-FREE, UNDER 500 CALORIES, VEGAN

Guacamole has many variations because this luscious condiment has a mild base. This version adds creamy yogurt, so the texture is velvety. If you prefer a chunkier guacamole, pulse the processor to combine the ingredients instead of puréeing or mashing the fruit by hand in a medium bowl, and stir in everything else.

1 ripe avocado, halved, peeled, and pitted

½ cup plain Greek yogurt

1 teaspoon minced garlic

Juice and zest of 1 lime

2 tablespoons chopped fresh basil

2 tablespoons chopped fresh cilantro

¼ teaspoon red pepper flakes

Sea salt

1. Put the avocado, yogurt, garlic, lime juice and zest, basil, cilantro, and red pepper flakes in a food processor and blend until smooth.

2. Season with salt and serve.

3. Store leftovers in the refrigerator for up to 3 days in a sealed container.

Substitution Tip: Try a plain coconut or soy yogurt instead of Greek yogurt to create a vegan version of this popular condiment. Or leave out the yogurt altogether for a classic guacamole.

PER SERVING: Calories: 99; Total fat: 7g; Saturated fat: 1g; Sodium: 21mg; Carbohydrates: 7g; Fiber: 3g; Protein: 5g

Chickpea–Cherry Tomato Salsa

SERVES 4 / PREP TIME: 15 MINUTES

30 MINUTES OR LESS, ALLERGEN-FREE, DAIRY-FREE, NUT-FREE, ONE POT, UNDER 500 CALORIES, VEGAN

Salsa can be mild or hot depending on the type and number of chiles used. The jalapeño pepper in this recipe is not considered to be an excessively hot pepper, but still contains enough capsaicin—which brings the heat—to tease the palate. Capsaicin has medicinal benefits like relieving arthritis pain, boosting the immune system, fighting heart disease, and supporting weight loss.

3 cups quartered cherry tomatoes

1 (15-ounce) can sodium-free chickpeas, drained and rinsed

1 yellow bell pepper, finely chopped

½ cup chopped sweet onion

½ jalapeño pepper, seeded and minced

¼ cup chopped fresh cilantro

1 teaspoon minced garlic

Juice and zest of 1 lime

Sea salt

1. In a large bowl, mix together the tomatoes, chickpeas, bell pepper, onion, jalapeño, cilantro, garlic, lime juice, and lime zest.

2. Season with salt and serve.

3. Store the salsa in a sealed container in the refrigerator for up to 4 days.

Variation Tip: Instead of chickpeas, lentils, black beans, or kidney beans would also be delicious in this fresh salsa. Use the same amount as you would chickpeas.

PER SERVING: Calories: 107; Total fat: 1g; Saturated fat: 0g; Sodium: 109mg; Carbohydrates: 22g; Fiber: 4g; Protein: 5g

Orange-Cilantro Vinaigrette

MAKES ¾ CUP / PREP TIME: 5 MINUTES

5 INGREDIENTS OR LESS, 30 MINUTES OR LESS, ALLERGEN-FREE, DAIRY-FREE, NUT-FREE, ONE POT, UNDER 500 CALORIES, VEGAN

Sweet orange and fresh cilantro can be the ideal finish to salads or as the liquid to cook fish in fancy foil or parchment packets. The touch of cayenne pepper adds heat without overpowering the other ingredients. You can use ruby red grapefruit if you enjoy a less sweet dressing; half of the large fruit should be a perfect amount for the recipe.

½ cup olive oil
Juice and zest of 1 orange
1 tablespoon apple
   cider vinegar
1 tablespoon chopped
   fresh cilantro
Pinch cayenne pepper
Sea salt
Freshly ground
   black pepper

1. In a small bowl, whisk together the oil, orange juice and zest, vinegar, cilantro, and cayenne pepper until well blended.

2. Season with salt and pepper and shake well before serving.

3. Store the dressing in the refrigerator in a sealed container for up to 2 weeks.

Craving Tip: The orange adds sweetness to any salad, so use on robust greens or crunchy vegetables rather than fruit-based recipes. This is just sweet enough to curb cravings for sugar.

PER SERVING (2 TABLESPOONS): Calories: 149; Total fat: 16g; Saturated fat: 2g; Sodium: 15mg; Carbohydrates: 1g; Fiber: 0g; Protein: 0g

Oil & Vinegar Dressing

MAKES ¾ CUP / PREP TIME: 5 MINUTES

5 INGREDIENTS OR LESS, 30 MINUTES OR LESS, ALLERGEN-FREE, DAIRY-FREE, NUT-FREE, ONE POT, UNDER 500 CALORIES, VEGAN

The result of combining oil and vinegar is called an emulsion. This is a fancy term for two unmixable liquids staying together due to a process or additional ingredient. The mustard in this recipe aids in the emulsification process, so do not leave it out. In the case of this dressing, the emulsification is not permanent; you will need to shake the container or whisk it again to create a vinaigrette that will coat your salads uniformly.

½ cup olive oil

¼ cup white wine or apple cider vinegar

2 teaspoons Dijon mustard

1 tablespoon chopped fresh herbs

½ teaspoon minced garlic

Sea salt

Freshly ground black pepper

1. In a small bowl, whisk together the oil, vinegar, mustard, herbs, and garlic until well blended.

2. Season with salt and pepper and shake well before serving.

3. Store the dressing in the refrigerator in a sealed container for up to 2 weeks.

Variation Tip: This is a base dressing—delicious on its own, but you can dress it up with different vinegars, herbs, or oils. Try balsamic vinegar for richness and depth and avocado oil for a lighter taste than olive oil.

PER SERVING (2 TABLESPOONS): Calories: 147; Total fat: 16g; Saturated fat: 2g; Sodium: 40mg; Carbohydrates: 0g; Fiber: 0g; Protein: 0g

Spinach-Lemon Hummus

SERVES 4 / PREP TIME: 15 MINUTES

30 MINUTES OR LESS, NUT-FREE, UNDER 500 CALORIES, VEGAN

Fresh citrus, smoky tahini, and pungent garlic are the base notes in this traditional Middle Eastern chickpea dip. The fresh spinach is chopped very finely and shows up as tiny green flecks. You can use hummus as a topping for proteins, in wraps, as a dip, or even stirred into soups for added flavor.

1 (15-ounce) can sodium-free chickpeas, drained and rinsed
1 cup fresh baby spinach
¼ cup tahini
Juice of 1 lemon
2 tablespoons olive oil
1 teaspoon minced garlic
¼ teaspoon ground cumin
Sea salt

1. Place the chickpeas, spinach, tahini, lemon juice, oil, garlic, and cumin in a food processor and pulse until the mixture is smooth.

2. Season with salt and serve.

3. Store in a sealed container for up to 1 week in the refrigerator.

Variation Tip: Hummus can be made with an incredible array of ingredients such as cauliflower, other legumes, pumpkin, kale, or sweet potato. Try different variations until you find your favorite combination.

PER SERVING: Calories: 205; Total fat: 15g; Saturated fat: 2g; Sodium: 136mg; Carbohydrates: 15g; Fiber: 2g; Protein: 6g

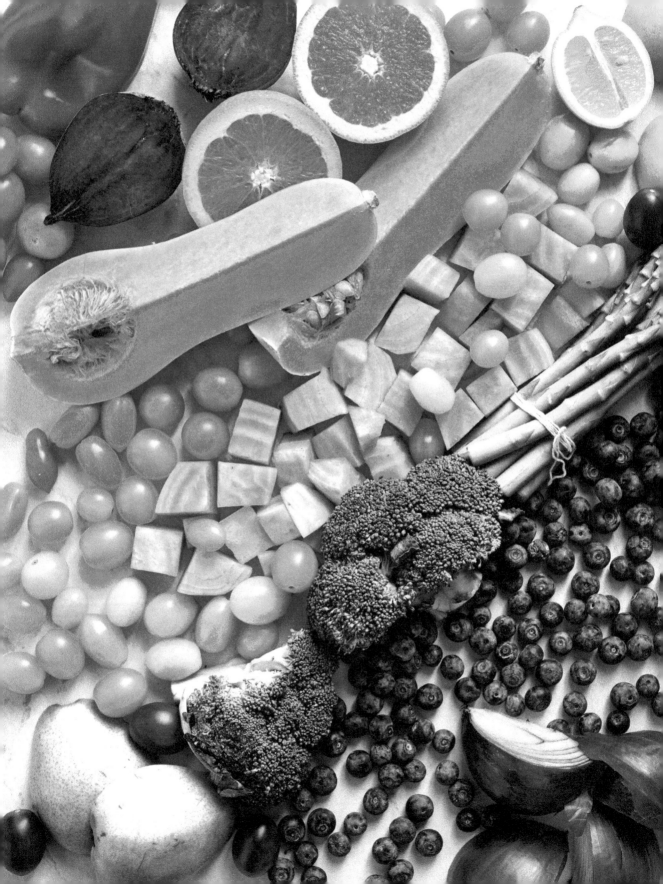

Measurement Conversions

	US STANDARD	US STANDARD (ounces)	Metric (approximate)
VOLUME EQUIVALENTS (LIQUID)	2 tablespoons	1 fl. oz.	30 mL
	¼ cup	2 fl. oz.	60 mL
	½ cup	4 fl. oz.	120 mL
	1 cup	8 fl. oz.	240 mL
	1½ cups	12 fl. oz.	355 mL
	2 cups or 1 pint	16 fl. oz.	475 mL
	4 cups or 1 quart	32 fl. oz.	1 L
	1 gallon	128 fl. oz.	4 L
VOLUME EQUIVALENTS (DRY)	⅛ teaspoon	———	0.5 mL
	¼ teaspoon	———	1 mL
	½ teaspoon	———	2 mL
	¾ teaspoon	———	4 mL
	1 teaspoon	———	5 mL
	1 tablespoon	———	15 mL
	¼ cup	———	59 mL
	⅓ cup	———	79 mL
	½ cup	———	118 mL
	⅔ cup	———	156 mL
	¾ cup	———	177 mL
	1 cup	———	235 mL
	2 cups or 1 pint	———	475 mL
	3 cups	———	700 mL
	4 cups or 1 quart	———	1 L
	½ gallon	———	2 L
	1 gallon	———	4 L
WEIGHT EQUIVALENTS	½ ounce	———	15 g
	1 ounce	———	30 g
	2 ounces	———	60 g
	4 ounces	———	115 g
	8 ounces	———	225 g
	12 ounces	———	340 g
	16 ounces or 1 pound	———	455 g

	FAHRENHEIT (F)	CELSIUS (C) (APPROXIMATE)
OVEN TEMPERATURES	250°F	120°C
	300°F	150°C
	325°F	180°C
	375°F	190°C
	400°F	200°C
	425°F	220°C
	450°F	230°C

References

Aird, T. P., R. W. Davies, and B. P. Carson. "Effects of Fasted vs Fed-State Exercise on Performance and Post-Exercise Metabolism: A Systematic Review and Meta-Analysis." *Scandinavian Journal of Medicine & Science in Sports* 28, no. 5 (2018): 1476–93.

Antoni, R., K. L. Johnston, A. L. Collins, and M. D. Robertson. "Intermittent v. Continuous Energy Restriction: Differential Effects on Postprandial Glucose and Lipid Metabolism Following Matched Weight Loss in Overweight/Obese Participants." *British Journal of Nutrition* 119, no. 5 (2018): 507–16.

Cağlayan, E. K., A. Y. Göçmen, and N. Delibas. "Effects of Long-Term Fasting on Female Hormone Levels: Ramadan Model." *Clinical and Experimental Obstetrics and Gynecology* 41 (2014): 17–19.

Campos-Nonato, I., L. Hernandez, and S. Barquera. "Effect of a High-Protein Diet Versus Standard-Protein Diet on Weight Loss and Biomarkers of Metabolic Syndrome: A Randomized Clinical Trial." *Obesity Facts* 10, no. 3 (2017): 238–51.

Chaouachi, A., J. B. Leiper, H. Chtourou, A. R. Aziz, and K. Chamari. "The Effects of Ramadan Intermittent Fasting on Athletic Performance: Recommendations for the Maintenance of Physical Fitness." *Journal of Sports Sciences* 30 suppl. 1 (2012): S53–73.

Cioffi, I., A. Evangelista, V. Ponzo, G. Ciccone, L. Soldati, L. Santarpia, F. Contaldo, et al. "Intermittent Versus Continuous Energy Restriction on Weight Loss and Cardiometabolic Outcomes: A Systematic Review and Meta-Analysis of Randomized Controlled Trials." *Journal of Translational Medicine* 16, no. 1 (2018): 371.

Erdem, Y., G. Ozkan, S. Ulusoy, M. Arici, U. Derici, S. Sengul, S. Sindel, et al. "The Effect of Intermittent Fasting on Blood Pressure Variability in Patients with Newly Diagnosed Hypertension or Prehypertension." *Journal of the American Society of Hypertension* 12, no. 1 (2018): 42–49.

Francis, L., J. Young, and J. Lara. "The Impact of Intermittent Fasting on Body Composition and Cardiovascular Biomarkers: A Systematic Review and Meta-Analysis." *Proceedings of the Nutrition Society* 76, no. OCE2 (2017).

Gabel, K., K. K. Hoddy, N. Haggerty, J. Song, C. M. Kroeger, J. F. Trepanowski, S. Panda, and K. A. Varady. "Effects of 8-Hour Time-Restricted Feeding on Body Weight and Metabolic Disease Risk Factors in Obese Adults: A Pilot Study." *Nutrition and Healthy Aging* 4, no. 4 (2018): 345–53.

Ganesan, K., Y. Habboush, and S. Sultan. "Intermittent Fasting: The Choice for a Healthier Lifestyle." *Cureus Journal of Medical Science* 10, no. 7 (2018): e2947.

Harris, L., A. McGarty, L. Hutchison, L. Ells, and C. Hankey. "Short-Term Intermittent Energy Restriction Interventions for Weight Management: A Systematic Review and Meta-Analysis." *Obesity Reviews* 19, no. 1 (2018): 1–13.

Harvie, M., and A. Howell. "Potential Benefits and Harms of Intermittent Energy Restriction and Intermittent Fasting Amongst Obese, Overweight and Normal Weight Subjects—a Narrative Review of Human and Animal Evidence." *Behavioural Sciences* 7, no. 1 (2017).

Harvie, M. N., M. Pegington, M. P. Mattson, J. Frystyk, B. Dillon, G. Evans, J. Cuzick, et al. "The Effects of Intermittent or Continuous Energy Restriction on Weight Loss and Metabolic Disease Risk Markers: A Randomized Trial in Young Overweight Women." *International Journal of Obesity* 35, no. 5 (2011): 714–27.

Institute of Medicine. *Dietary Reference Intakes for Water, Potassium, Sodium, Chloride, and Sulfate.* Washington DC: The National Academies Press, 2005.

Isganaitis, E., and R. H. Lustig. "Fast Food, Central Nervous System Insulin Resistance, and Obesity." *Arteriosclerosis, Thrombosis, and Vascular Biology* 25, no. 12 (2005): 2451–62.

Jamshed, H., R. A. Beyl, D. L. Della Manna, E. S. Yang, E. Ravussin, and C. M. Peterson. "Early Time-Restricted Feeding Improves 24-Hour Glucose Levels and Affects Markers of the Circadian Clock, Aging, and Autophagy in Humans." *Nutrients* 11, no. 6 (2019).

Larsson, C. A., B. Gullberg, L. Rastam, and U. Lindblad. "Salivary Cortisol Differs with Age and Sex and Shows Inverse Associations with WHR in Swedish Women: A Cross-Sectional Study." *BMC Endocrine Disorders* 9 (2009): 16.

Leidy, H. J., P. M. Clifton, A. Astrup, T. P. Wycherley, M. S. Westerterp-Plantenga, N. D. Luscombe-Marsh, S. C. Woods, and R. D. Mattes. "The Role of Protein in Weight Loss and Maintenance." *American Journal of Clinical Nutrition* 101, no. 6 (2015): 1320S–29S.

Lessan, N., and T. Ali. "Energy Metabolism and Intermittent Fasting: The Ramadan Perspective." *Nutrients* 11, no. 5 (2019).

Mahnaz, Y., M. Amirzargar, N. Amirzargar, and M. Dadashpour. "Does Ramadan Fasting Have Any Effects on Menstrual Cycles?" *Iranian Journal of Reproductive Medicine* 11, no. 2 (2013): 145–50.

Malinowski, B., K. Zalewska, A. Wesierska, M. M. Sokolowska, M. Socha, G. Liczner, K. Pawlak-Osińska, and M. Wicinski. "Intermittent Fasting in Cardiovascular Disorders—an Overview." *Nutrients* 11, no. 3 (2019).

Mindikoglu, A. L., A. R. Opekun, S. K. Gagan, and S. Devaraj. "Impact of Time-Restricted Feeding and Dawn-to-Sunset Fasting on Circadian Rhythm, Obesity, Metabolic Syndrome, and Nonalcoholic Fatty Liver Disease." *Gastroenterology Research and Practice* (2017): 3932491.

Mitchell, S. J., M. Bernier, J. A. Mattison, M. A. Aon, T. A. Kaiser, R. M. Anson, Y. Ikeno, et al. "Daily Fasting Improves Health and Survival in Male Mice Independent of Diet Composition and Calories." *Cell Metabolism* 29, no. 1 (2019): 221–28 e3.

Moro, T., G. Tinsley, A. Bianco, G. Marcolin, Q. F. Pacelli, G. Battaglia, A. Palma, et al. "Effects of Eight Weeks of Time-Restricted Feeding (16/8) on Basal Metabolism, Maximal Strength, Body Composition, Inflammation, and Cardiovascular Risk Factors in Resistance-Trained Males." *Journal of Translational Medicine* 14, no. 1 (Oct. 13, 2016): 290.

Muoio, D. M. "Metabolic Inflexibility: When Mitochondrial Indecision Leads to Metabolic Gridlock." *Cell* 159, no. 6 (2014): 1253–62.

Paoli, A., G. Tinsley, A. Bianco, and T. Moro. "The Influence of Meal Frequency and Timing on Health in Humans: The Role of Fasting." *Nutrients* 11, no. 4 (2019).

Patterson, R. E., G. A. Laughlin, A. Z. LaCroix, S. J. Hartman, L. Natarajan, C. M. Senger, M. E. Martinez, et al. "Intermittent Fasting and Human Metabolic Health." *Journal of the Academy of Nutrition and Dietetics* 115, no. 8 (Aug 2015): 1203–12.

Patterson, R. E., and Dorothy D. Sears. "Metabolic Effects of Intermittent Fasting." *Annual Review of Nutrition* 37 (2017): 371–93.

Prochaska, J. O., S. Butterworth, C. A. Redding, V. Burden, N. Perrin, M. Leo, M. Flaherty-Robb, and J. M. Prochaska. "Initial Efficacy of MI, TTM Tailoring and HRI's with Multiple Behaviors for Employee Health Promotion." *Preventative Medicine* 46, no. 3 (2008): 226–31.

Ravussin, E., R. A. Beyl, E. Poggiogalle, D. S. Hsia, and C. M. Peterson. "Early Time-Restricted Feeding Reduces Appetite and Increases Fat Oxidation but Does Not Affect Energy Expenditure in Humans." *Obesity* 27, no. 8 (2019): 1244–54.

Rohit V., Y. P. Balhara, and C. S. Gupta. "Gender Differences in Stress Response: Role of Developmental and Biological Determinants." *Indian Journal of Psychiatry* 20, no. 1 (2011): 4–10.

Santos, H. O., and R. C. O. Macedo. "Impact of Intermittent Fasting on the Lipid Profile: Assessment Associated with Diet and Weight Loss." *Clinical Nutrition ESPEN* 24 (2018): 14–21.

Scheer, F. A., C. J. Morris, and S. A. Shea. "The Internal Circadian Clock Increases Hunger and Appetite in the Evening Independent of Food Intake and Other Behaviors." *Obesity* 21, no. 3 (2013): 421–3.

Seimon, R., J. A. Roekenesa, J. Zibellinia, B. Zhua, A. A. Gibsona, A. P. Hills, R. E. Wood, N. A. King, N. M. Byrne, A. Sainsbury. "Do Intermittent Diets Provide Physiological Benefits over Continuous Diets for Weight Loss? A Systematic Review of Clinical Trials." *Molecular and Cellular Endocrinology* 418 (2015): 153–72.

Stockman, M. C., D. Thomas, J. Burke, and C. M. Apovian. "Intermittent Fasting: Is the Wait Worth the Weight?" *Current Obesity Reports* 7, no. 2 (June 2018): 172–85.

Sutton, E. F., R. Beyl, K. S. Early, W. T. Cefalu, E. Ravussin, and C. M. Peterson. "Early Time-Restricted Feeding Improves Insulin Sensitivity, Blood Pressure, and Oxidative Stress Even without Weight Loss in Men with Prediabetes." *Cell Metabolism* 27, no. 6 (June 5, 2018): 1212–21 e3.

Tinsley, G. M., M. L. Moore, A. J. Graybeal, A. Paoli, Y. Kim, J. U. Gonzales, J. R. Harry, et al. "Time-Restricted Feeding Plus Resistance Training in Active Females: A Randomized Trial." *American Journal of Clinical Nutrition* 110, no. 3 (Sep. 1, 2019): 628–40.

Trepanowski, J. F., C. M. Kroeger, A. Barnosky, M. C. Klempel, S. Bhutani, K. K. Hoddy, K. Gabel, et al. "Effect of Alternate Day Fasting on Weight Loss, Weight Maintenance, and Cardioprotection Among Metabolically Healthy Obese Adults: A Randomized Clinical Trial." *JAMA Internal Medicine* 177, no. 7 (2017): 930–38.

Wegman, M. P., M. H. Guo, and M. L. Brantly. "Practicality of Intermittent Fasting in Humans and Its Effect on Oxidative Stress and Genes Related to Aging and Metabolism." *Rejuvenation Research* 18 no. 2 (2015): 162–172. NCBI.NLM.NIH.gov/pmc/articles /PMC4403246.

Westerterp-Plantenga, M. S. "The Significance of Protein in Food Intake and Body Weight Regulation." *Current Opinion in Clinical Nutrition and Metabolic Care* 6 (2003): 635–38.

Index

Acknowledgments

This being my fourth print publication, I am increasingly aware of the need to make the most of this section, if for no other reason than the fact that I have a number of people in my life who are deeply deserving of acknowledgment.

They know who they are, and yet sadly, not all of them are still with me.

One in particular is my dear lifelong friend Josh, who would have been especially fascinated by this book. A journal-published mental health nutrition researcher and one of my best friends, Josh was always ahead of the curve when it came to an interest in food and a passion for dietary trends and science. I can say with utter certainty that he would have been quite intrigued by intermittent fasting and may have even been dabbling in it without telling me.

Josh's fascination with nutrition went all the way back to our teenage years, when my main interest was which chocolate bar or bag of candy I was getting from the high school vending machine that day. He was more likely to be interested in which vegetables were being served for dinner that night. Despite being two years my junior, he was wise and kind beyond his time and taught me a great deal about what it meant to be a good person who is committed to their craft. And yeah, playing video games together was fun, too.

At the time of his passing, on February 5, 2015, I had not yet started my private practice and had no website, no blog, no social media presence—and certainly no published books. Four-plus years later, as these words land on the page of my fourth piece of authorship, I fulfill an eternal promise to a friend that I would take him with me along for the ride.

Here's to you, dude.

About the Authors

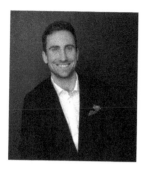

Andy De Santis, RD, MPH, is a registered dietitian, speaker, and multibook author from Toronto, Canada. He operates a private dietetics practice focused on customized nutrition solutions for people who deal with a wide array of health concerns, and prides himself on providing exceptional and charismatic care to his clients. Andy has been featured in local newspapers, in magazines, and on television. He is never afraid to offer his views on important topics in the field of nutrition. When he isn't helping people in a one-on-one setting, Andy loves creating hard-hitting content with a lighthearted twist on his personal blog AndyTheRD.com and various social media accounts, including Instagram (@AndyTheRD).

Michelle Anderson is the author and ghostwriter of more than 30 cookbooks focused on healthy diets and delicious food. She worked as a professional chef for more than 25 years, honing her craft overseas in North Africa and all over Ontario, Canada, in fine restaurants. She worked as a corporate executive chef for Rational Canada for four years, collaborating with her international counterparts and consulting in kitchens all over Southern Ontario and in the United States. Michelle ran her own catering company and personal chef business, and was also a wedding cake designer. Her focus was food as medicine, using wholesome, quality field-to-fork ingredients in vibrant, visually impactful dishes. Michelle lives in Temiskaming Shores, Ontario, Canada, with her husband, two sons, two Newfoundland dogs, and three cats.

CPSIA information can be obtained
at www.ICGtesting.com
Printed in the USA
LVHW020739190420
653872LV00001B/1

9 781646 115709